Current Cardiovascular Therapy

Arturo Evangelista
Christoph A. Nienaber
Editors

Juan Carlos Kaski
Series Editor

Pharmacotherapy in Aortic Disease

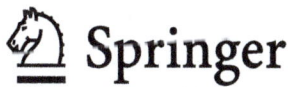 Springer

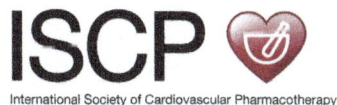

Editors

Arturo Evangelista, MD, FESC
Imaging Cardiac Department
Aortic Diseases Unit
Vall d'hebrón University
Hospital
Barcelona
Spain

Christoph A. Nienaber, MD, PhD
Heart Center Rostock
Rostock School of Medicine
University Hospital Rostock
Rostock
Germany

ISBN 978-3-319-09554-7   ISBN 978-3-319-09555-4   (eBook)
DOI 10.1007/978-3-319-09555-4
Springer Cham Heidelberg New York Dordrecht London

Library of Congress Control Number: 2014956265

Printed on acid-free paper

Springer is part of Springer Science+Business Media (www.springer.com)

Preface

Aortic diseases have classically been studied from a surgical point of view. Recently, considerable progress has been made in their diagnosis and understanding of their pathophysiology and evolution, mainly due to advent of imaging techniques. Despite the lack of symptoms in stable conditions, most aortic diseases have a high morbidity and mortality. In advanced phase of the disease, new therapeutic strategies such as endovascular treatment or surgical techniques have appeared to improve conventional surgery. However, until the last decade, most aortic diseases were only medically treated with control of cardiovascular risk factors and beta-blockers in an attempt to reduce aortic wall stress by reducing blood pressure and heart rate. Nevertheless, in recent years different studies have demonstrated the benefit of new treatments with subsequent changes in the natural history of these diseases.

The aim of this book is to provide an update on the medical treatment of the aorta diseases. To this end, leading aorta experts have made a critical, in-depth analysis of the recent evidences on medical treatment of different aortic disease entities. Both basic research studies and clinical trials discussed in this book serve as a base for improving therapeutic management, delaying the need for surgery and prolonging survival in these patients.

Barcelona, Spain   Arturo Evangelista, MD, FESC

Series Preface

Cardiovascular pharmacotherapy is of fundamental importance for the successful management of patients with cardiovascular diseases. Appropriate therapeutic decisions require a proper understanding of the disease and a thorough knowledge of the pharmacological agents available for clinical use. The issue is complicated by the existence of large numbers of agents with subtle differences in their mode of action and efficacy and the existence of national and international guidelines, which sometimes fail to deliver a clear cut message. Aggressive marketing techniques from pharma industry, financial issues at local, regional or national levels, and time constraints make it difficult for the practitioner to – at times – be absolutely certain as to whether drug selection is absolutely appropriate. The International Society of Cardiovascular Pharmacotherapy (ISCP) aims at supporting evidence based, rational pharmacotherapy worldwide. The present book series represents one of its vital educational tools. This series aims at contributing independent, balanced and sound information to help the busy practitioner to identify the appropriate pharmacological tools to deliver rational therapies. Topics in the series include all major cardiovascular scenarios and the books are edited and authored by experts in their fields. The books are intended for a wide range of healthcare professionals and particularly for younger consultants and physicians in training. All aspects of pharma cotherapy are tackled in the series in a concise and practical fashion. The books in the ISCP series provide a unique set of guidelines and examples that will prove valuable for patient management. They clearly articulate many of the dilemmas clinicians face when working to deliver sound therapies to their patients. The series will most certainly be a useful reference for those seeking to deliver evidence based, practical and successful cardiovascular pharmacotherapy.

Juan Carlos Kaski, DSc, DM (Hons),
MD, FRCP, FESC, FACC, FAHA

Contents

Contents

Contributors

Damiano Baldassarre Centro Cardiologico Monzino, IRCCS, Milan, Italy

Dipartimento di Scienze Farmacologiche e BiomolecolariUniversità di Milano, Milan, Italy

Ciro Bancone Cardiac Surgery Unit, Department of Cardiothoracic Sciences, Monaldi Hospital, University of Naples II, Naples, Italy

Eduardo Bossone, MD, PhD Heart Department, University Hospital "Scuola Medica Salernitana", Salerno, Italy

Claire Bouleti Centre National Maladies Rares Syndrome de Marfan et apparentés, INSERM U1148 (LVTS), Paris, France

Marianna Buonocore Cardiac Surgery School, Department of Cardiothoracic Sciences, University of Naples II, Naples, Italy

Rodolfo Citro, MD, PhD Heart Department, University Hospital "Scuola Medica Salernitana", Salerno, Italy

Heart DepartmentUniversity Hospital "Scuola Medica Salernitana", Salerno, Italy

Alessandro Della Corte, MD, PhD Cardiac Surgery Unit, Department of Cardiothoracic Sciences, Monaldi Hospital, University of Naples II, Naples, Italy

Arturo Evangelista, MD, FESC Division of Cardiology, Hospital Universitari Vall d'Hebron, Barcelona, Spain

Francesco Ferrara, MD, PhD Heart Department, University Hospital "Scuola Medica Salernitana", Salerno, Italy

Valentina Galuppo, MD Division of Cardiology, Hospital Universitari Vall d'Hebron, Barcelona, Spain

Guillaume Jondeau Centre National Maladies Rares Syndrome de Marfan et apparentés, INSERM U1148 (LVTS), Université Paris 7, AP-HP Hopital Bichat, Paris, France

Jean-Baptiste Michel INSERM U1148 (LVTS), Hopital Bichat, Paris, France

Olivier Milleron Centre National Maladies Rares Syndrome de Marfan et apparentés, INSERM U1148 (LVTS), AP-HP Hopital Bichat, Paris, France

Christoph A. Nienaber, MD, PhD Heart Center Rostock, University of Rostock, Rostock, Germany

Mauro Pepi Centro Cardiologico Monzino, IRCCS, Milan, Italy

Gisela Teixido-Tura, MD, PhD Division of Cardiology, Hospital Universitari Vall d'Hebron, Barcelona, Spain

Chapter 1
Aortic Atherosclerosis as an Embolic Source

Damiano Baldassarre and Mauro Pepi

Clinical Aspects

Cardioembolism

Stroke is the third leading cause of death in several industrial countries and cardiogenic embolism accounts for 15–30 % of ischaemic strokes [1–5]. The diagnosis of a cardioembolic source of stroke is frequently uncertain and relies on the identification of a potential cardiac source of embolism in the absence of significant autochthonous cerebrovascular occlusive disease. In this regard, echocardiography (either transthoracic – TTE or Transoesophageal – TEE) serves as a cornerstone in the evaluation and diagnosis of these patients [6, 7].

Cardioembolic stroke is a heterogeneous entity, since a variety of cardiac conditions can predispose to cerebral embolism. These cardiac conditions may be classified as major, minor or

D. Baldassarre
Centro Cardiologico Monzino, IRCCS, Milan, Italy

Dipartimento di Scienze Farmacologiche e Biomolecolari,
Università di Milano, Milan, Italy

M. Pepi (✉)
Centro Cardiologico Monzino, IRCCS, Milan, Italy
e-mail: mauro.pepi@ccfm.it

A. Evangelista, C.A. Nienaber (eds.), *Pharmacotherapy in Aortic Disease*, Current Cardiovascular Therapy, Vol. 7, DOI 10.1007/978-3-319-09555-4_1,
© Springer International Publishing Switzerland 2015

uncertain risk. The indications for and role of ultrasound techniques in these diseases are not well defined. Moreover, from a pathological point of view cardioembolic sources of embolism may be classified into three distinct categories: cardiac lesions that have a propensity for thrombus formation [i.e. thrombus formation in the left atrial appendage in patients with atrial fibrillation (AF)], cardiac masses (i.e. cardiac tumours, vegetations, thrombi, aortic atherosclerotic plaques) and passageways within the heart serving as conduits for paradoxical embolization (i.e. patent foramen ovale).

Aortic Atherosclerosis as an Embolic Source

Aortic atherosclerosis is inserted in major cardiovascular conditions predisposing to cerebral or peripheral embolism. Because of the large diameter of the vessel, even very large atherosclerotic and/or thrombosed plaques protruding into the lumen usually do not associate with aorta occlusion. So, even if advanced atherosclerotic manifestations may include atheroma, fibroatheroma and complex atheroma with surface erosions and luminal thrombi, the main clinical significance of aortic plaques lies in their embolic potentials [8]. Atherosclerosis may also contribute to the development of aortic aneurysms [9].

Aortic plaques are a source of two types of emboli: thromboemboli and atheroemboli.

Even if in both instances there is arterio-arterial embolism (i.e. embolisation from the aorta to its branches), the two types of problems differ in the size and content of emboli, in the rate of occurrence, and in their clinical manifestations, prognosis, and treatment [10, 11].

Thromboemboli

In thromboembolism there is typically an abrupt release of a solitary or a few large emboli containing fragments of a thrombus that usually derives from complex (large and mobile) atheromatous aortic plaques. Being relatively large, this type of embolus tends to occlude medium to large arteries, thus leading to severe ischaemia of target organs [12]. From a clinical point of view, aortic thromboembolism may be associated with sudden onset of serious signs and symptoms in a large vascular territory, which may cause stroke, transient ischaemic attacks (TIAs), myocardial infarction, renal or splenic infarcts, and other forms of peripheral thromboembolism.

Atheroemboli

Atheroemboli are composed of cholesterol crystals. They are usually smaller than thromboemboli and tend to occlude just small arteries and arterioles. The end-organ damage associated with this type of embolism may be due to both mechanical blood flow reduction and an inflammatory response. Atheroembolism is often characterised by a large number of small emboli (showers of microemboli) occurring in recurrent waves. This type of embolism may cause the blue toe syndrome, new or worsening renal failure, gut ischaemia, confusion, memory loss, etc. Clinically, atheroembolism is much less frequent that thromboembolism.

Both types of embolism may occur spontaneously; however, there is evidence suggesting that they may occur also as a consequence of an aortic iatrogenic procedure such as arteriography, intra-aortic balloon placement, percutaneous intervention, major vessel surgery, or thrombolytic therapy [13–26]. Large atherosclerotic plaques and intraluminal thrombi of the aorta may increase the risk of embolic stroke during manipulation of guidewires and catheters [27]. Plaque disruption due to these procedures may significantly increase the morbidity and mortality of aortic interventions such as transcatheter aortic valve insertion [28].

According to brain magnetic resonance imaging (MRI) or ultrasonographic procedures such as transcranial Doppler ultrasonography, after iatrogenic plaque disruption, clinically overt aortic embolism is much less frequent than the silent one [29].

Clinical Presentation

Clinical consequences of aortic embolisation may vary considerably, from a complete absence of symptoms to acute multiorgan failure such as new to worsening renal failure or cutaneous involvement [30]. The clinical manifestation of aortic embolism depends (1) on the location of the aortic plaque forming the embolus, (2) on the atherosclerotic or thrombotic nature of the embolus (atheroembolus or thromboembolus), and (3) on the arterial district that the embolus occludes.

Aortic Arch Atheroma and Ischaemic Stroke

According to intraoperative ultrasonographic [31], TEE [14, 32–36], and autopsy studies [37, 38] aortic arch atheroma is a risk factor for ischaemic stroke. In particular, in about one-third of patients with otherwise unexplained stroke, complicated atherosclerotic plaques with a thickness ≥ 4 mm in the aortic arch proximal to the origin of the left subclavian artery, represent an independent risk factor for stroke and systemic embolism similar to atrial fibrillation and severe atherosclerosis of the carotid arteries [38].

In these patients, even if treated with antiplatelet drug, the 1-year risk of recurrent ischaemic stroke is ≈ 11 %, and the 1-, 2- and 3-year risk of a combined vascular event (ischaemic stroke, MI, peripheral event, or vascular death), is 20, 36, and 50 %, respectively [39, 40].

The risk of new ischaemic stroke and that of new combined vascular events were 3.8 (95 % CI 1.8–7.8, $P \leq 0.002$) and 3.5 (95 % CI 2.1–5.9, $P \leq 0.001$), respectively, independent of carotid stenosis, atrial fibrillation, peripheral artery disease, or other risk factors [39]. The presence of an aortic arch plaque is also an independent predictor of recurrent strokes, MI and vascular death [13, 41–43].

Aortic Arch Atheroma Evolution Over Time

The morphological natural evolution of the aortic arch atheroma is a dynamic process with formation and resolution of mobile components occurring frequently over the same period. Sen et al. [44], described aortic arch atheroma progression in 29 % of patients and regression in about 9 %. Montgomery et al. [45], over a mean of 1 year, reported progression in 23 % and regression in 10 %. Pistavos et al. [46], in patients with familial hypercholesterolaemia taking pravastatin reported progression over 2 years in 19 % of patients and regression in 38 %. Geraci and Weinberger [47] noted a progression rate of 19 % and a regression rate of 18 % over a mean of 7.7 months. Importantly, aortic arch atheroma progression in patients with stroke/TIA has been associated with a higher rate of vascular events [48].

Location of the Aortic Plaque Forming the Embolus

Usually, the more distal the location of aortic plaque is, the lower the number of aortic branch which can be potentially affected. For example, lower extremities arterial circulation may receive emboli from any portion of the aorta; the splanchnic and renal arteries are usually affected by emboli from the thoracic aorta or from the proximal part of the abdominal aorta whereas coronary, cerebral, and upper extremity arteries usually receive emboli just from plaques in the ascending aorta and in the aortic arch. Skin embolism may arise from plaque in any portion of the thoraco-abdominal aorta. Despite this, a number of evidences has now shown that protruding atheromas in ascending aorta [31, 49, 50], in the aortic arch [32, 50–54], in the thoracic aorta [34, 55, 56] and mural aortic thrombi [57] are all direct causes not only of peripheral atheroembolism but also of cerebral atheroembolism which may increase the risk for ischaemic stroke.

Therefore, even if emboli forming from plaques in the descending thoracic aorta may embolise retrogradely into the aortic arch vessels during aortic flow reversal in diastole [58], usually the more distal the location of aortic plaque is, the lower is the number of aortic branches which can be potentially affected.

Risk Factors for the Development of Aortic Atheroma Forming the Embolus

Both types of aorta embolisms (thromboembolism and atheroembolism) occur in the general context of atherosclerosis. Indeed, conventional (sex, age, heredity, dyslipidemia, diabetes mellitus, hypertension, sedentary lifestyle, smoking, and endothelial dysfunction) and non-conventional (elevated levels of inflammatory markers, e.g. serum C-reactive protein, homocysteine, or lipoprotein) atherosclerosis risk factors concur in the development of aortic atheroma [59, 60]. The risk for embolic complications is increased in the presence of large (≥ 4 mm) or complex aortic plaques (such as plaques containing mobile thrombi or ulcerations) [61]. Calcified plaques are more stable and less prone to rupture [61–63], whereas noncalcified plaques, plaques with a larger lipid core or rich in macrophages and plaque with thin fibrous cap are more prone to disruption or rupture and more likely to result in embolic syndromes. In addition, beside iatrogenic manipulation, the likelihood of embolisation is also increased in the presence of inflammation, arterial rheological change due to hypertension, plaque haemorrhage, and aneurysms.

Nature of the Embolus

Although the thromboembolism and atheroembolism share the same risk factors, they are not mutually exclusive, and one patient may experience both type of embolisms at the same time.

In thromboembolism, clot fragments usually originate from the surface of stage VI lesions and tend to embolise to the distant circulation. From a clinical point of view, the result of this macro-embolism is a sudden onset of signs and symptoms, often severe, related to occlusion of medium to large arteries (e.g. coronary, cerebral, renal or popliteal). Due to the abrupt occlusion of a large vascular bed, the onset of symptoms often corresponds to a maximum organ deficit.

In atheroembolism, instead, cholesterol crystals, originating from the lipid core of an aortic atherosclerotic plaque, are released as repetitive waves of microemboli (showers of emboli). Atheroembolism is clinically much less prevalent than thromboembolism [64] and, typically, occlude arterioles with diameter not greater than 200 μm. The cholesterol embolisation syndrome is not easy to recognise. In fact, its clinical manifestation is often an inflammatory reaction in the affected vascular district and a combination of nonspecific acute inflammatory response (fever, malaise, hypereosinophilia, eosinophiluria, and elevated erythrocyte sedimentation rate) and organ-specific manifestations [65, 66].

Diagnosis and Severity Classification of Aortic Atheroma (TTE, TEE, CT, MRI)

Methods of imaging the aortic arch to detect and/or measure a plaque include: Transthoracic Echocardiography, Transoesophageal Echocardiography, Epiaortic Ultrasonography, Contrast Aortography, Magnetic Resonance Imaging, and Computed Tomography. Table 1.1 summarises advantages and disadvantages of the different imaging modalities.

Transthoracic Echocardiography (TTE)

TTE allows assessment of the aortic root and the proximal ascending aorta but cannot adequately image aortic arch plaques [67, 68]. However, echocardiographic evaluation of the aorta is a routine part of the standard echocardiographic examination. Although TTE is not the technique of choice for overall assessment of the aorta, it is useful for the diagnosis

TABLE 1.1 Imaging modalities in the evaluation of aortic atheroma

Imaging modality	Setting (labs vs intensive care units, interventional or operating room)	Feasibility (selective criteria; renal function)	Accuracy in wall evaluation and non mobile atheroma	Accuracy in wall evaluation and mobile atheroma	Panoramic imaging and data of the aortic vessels	Cost	Invasiveness	Contrast agents
TTE	All	++++	++	+	+	+	−	−
TEE	All	++++	++++	++++	++	++	+	−
Cardiac CT	RX laboratory	+++	++++	+	++++	+++	−	+
Cardiac MR	RX laboratory	+++	+++	++	++++	++++	−	+
Angiography	Interventional	+	+	+	+++	++++	++++	+
Epiaortic Echo	Operating room	+	++++	++++	+	++++	++	−

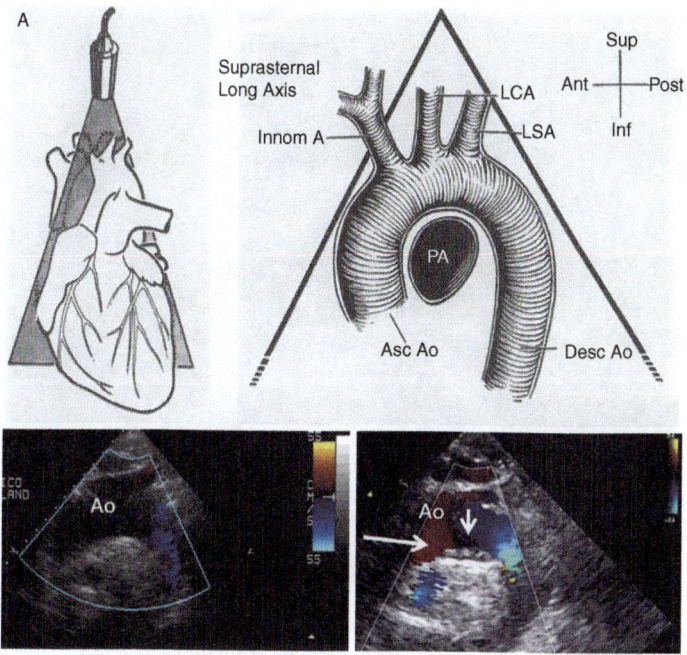

FIGURE 1.1 Schematic representation of the aortic arch as seen by transthoracic echo from the suprasternal view. The true echo images (*bottom*) show on the left a normal appearance of the arch and an example of on atheroma at the level of the ventral part of the arch (*arrow*)

and follow-up of some segments of the aorta. TTE is one of the techniques most used to measure proximal aortic segments in clinical practice [69, 70]. The long-axis view affords the best opportunity for measuring aortic root diameters by taking advantage of the superior axial image resolution. Of paramount importance for evaluation of the thoracic aorta is the suprasternal view (Figs. 1.1 and 1.2). This view primarily depicts the aortic arch and the three major supra-aortic vessels (innominate, left carotid, and left subclavian arteries), with variable lengths of the descending and, to a lesser degree, ascending aorta. Although this view may be obstructed, particularly in patients with emphysema or short, wide necks, it should be systematically sought if aortic disease is evaluated.

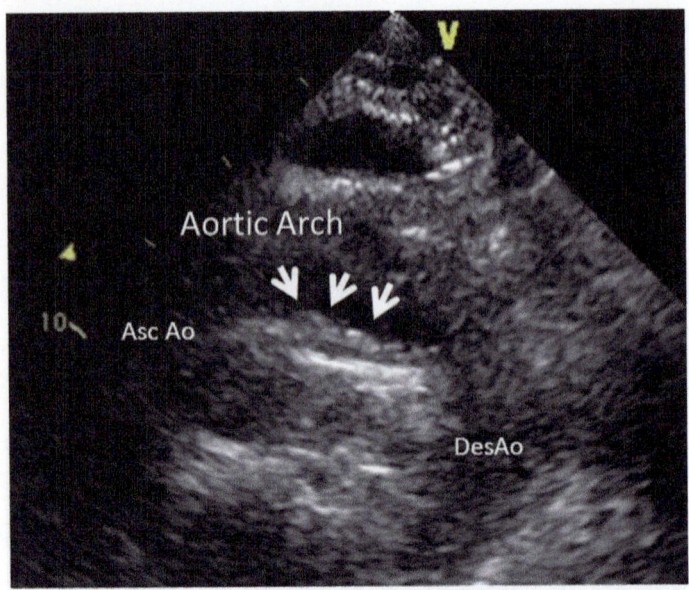

FIGURE 1.2 Example of an atheroma of the aortic arch (*arrows*) visualized from the suprasternal view by transthoracic echo

From this window, aortic coarctation can be visualised and functionally evaluated by continuous-wave Doppler; a persistent ductus arteriosus may also be identifiable by colour Doppler. Dilatation and aneurysm, plaque, calcification, thrombus, or dissection membranes are detectable if image quality is sufficient. A systematic comparison of harmonic TTE and TEE made to detect aortic plaques and thrombi revealed high sensitivity for the detection of aortic arch atheromas protruding ≥4 mm into the lumen [2]. However, the entire thoracic descending aorta is not well visualised by TTE.

Transoesophageal Echocardiography (TEE)

TEE allows us not only to assess plaque mobility, ulceration, and composition [71], but also to obtain detailed information on the anatomic relationship between the plaque location and the origin of the large arterial branches [12, 25, 32, 72–76].

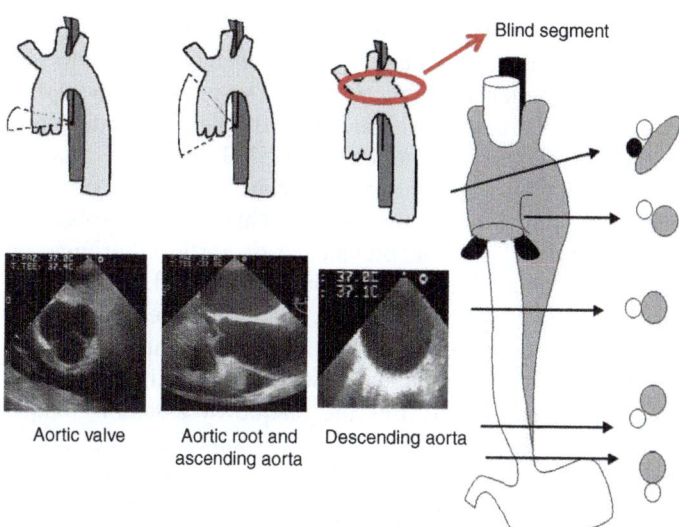

FIGURE 1.3 Schematic representation of the thoracic aorta and relative position of the transoesophageal echo probe inside the oesophagus. The entire aorta may be visualized by gentle rotation of the probe anteriorly or posteriorly. *Bottom*: corresponding TEE examples of the short axis of the aortic valve (*bottom left*), long axis of the proximal and ascending aorta (*bottom middle*) and short axis of the descending aorta (*bottom right*). The *red circle* and *arrow* show the blind segment of the aortic arch due to the interposition of the left bronchus

Beside the possibility of structural damage, other limitations associated with this diagnostic technique include the need for conscious sedation and patient cooperation for swallowing the probe, both quite difficult in patients with stroke [71]. In addition, due to the shadow associated with the tracheal air column near the origin of the innominate artery, which masks a portion of the ascending aorta when monoplanar and biplanar probes are used, an estimated 2 % of plaques are missed [77]. The use of multiplanar probes may reduce this problem [78] (Fig. 1.3).

The presence of detectable atherosclerotic plaques in the aorta indicates the presence of atherosclerotic disease and is a possible source of embolism [12]. Aortic atheromas are characterised by irregular intimal thickening of at least 2 mm, with increased echogenicity. They often have superimposed mobile components, mainly thrombi. The morphology of atheromatous plaques is dynamic, with frequent formation and resolution of mobile components [45]. TEE is the imaging modality of choice for diagnosing aortic atheromas. It provides higher-resolution images than TTE and has good inter-observer reproducibility [79]. The prevalence of aortic atheromas on TEE varies depending on the population studied. In a community-based TEE study [80], aortic atheromas were present in 51 % of the population over 45 years, being complex in 7.6 %. Atheroma prevalence increased with age, smoking, and pulse pressure. TEE characterises the plaque by assessing plaque thickness, ulceration, calcification and superimposed mobile thrombi, thereby determining the embolic potential of each plaque. The advantages of TEE over other non-invasive modalities include its ability to assess the mobility of plaque in real time. The French Aortic Plaque in Stroke group showed that increasing plaque thickness of ≥ 4 mm is associated with a significantly increased embolic risk [39]. They used TEE to characterise aortic arch plaque thickness in 331 patients older than 60 years with stroke. Increasing plaque thickness was associated with an increased risk of embolic events. The odds ratio for aortic arch plaque <1 mm and stroke was 1.0. The odds ratio was 3.9 for plaque between 1 and 3.9 mm thick and 13.8 for plaques >4 mm thick. The presence of mobile lesions (thrombi) superimposed on aortic atheromas has been recognized to imply a high embolic risk. Other characteristics of the lesions seen on TEE, such as ulceration ≥ 2 mm in aortic plaques and no calcified plaques, were also associated with a higher risk of stroke [81]. Thus, atherosclerotic plaques are defined as complex in the presence of protruding atheromas of 4 mm in thickness, mobile debris, or the presence of plaque ulceration, and defined as simple if the plaques lack these morphological features (Fig. 1.4).

A grading system for severity of atherosclerosis in the thoracic aorta has been proposed by Montgomery. Grade I = normal or minimal intimal thickening; Grade II: extensive

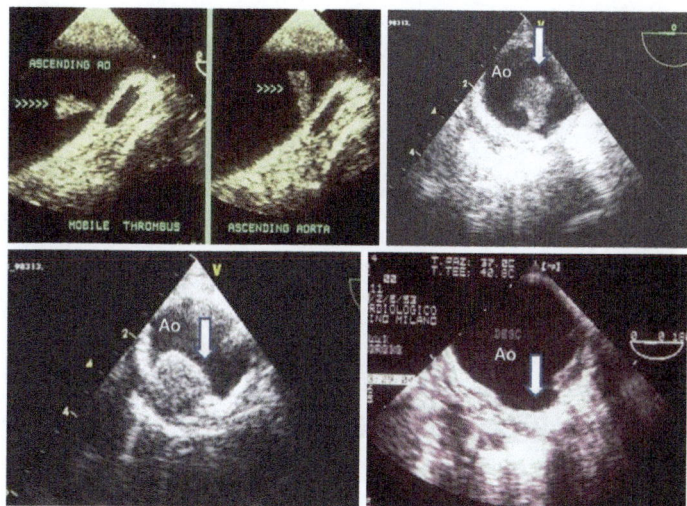

FIGURE 1.4 Examples of TEE images of different cases of thoracic aorta pathologies that may be correlated to embolic events. *Top left*: TEE of the distal ascending aorta showing a mobile thrombus attached to aortic wall (*arrows* indicate the mobility of the thrombus in two different frames). *Top right*: TEE of the descending aorta. In this short axis a very large protruding thrombus attached to a large aortic plaque is clearly detected. *Bottom left*: TEE of the descending thoracic aorta. Large protruding atheroma of the aortic wall. *Bottom right*: TEE of the descending thoracic aorta: large ulcerated plaque with a crater like appearance (*arrow*)

intimal thickening; Grade III = atheroma <5 mm; Grade IV = atheroma ≥5 mm; Grade V = mobile lesion (Fig. 1.5).

Two recent community-based studies found no association between aortic atheromas and future stroke [59, 80]. An alternative explanation is that atheromatous plaque is merely a marker for diffuse atherosclerosis that predisposes patients to systemic embolism by other cardiovascular mechanisms. The embolic potential of atherosclerotic aortic lesions during invasive procedures or during open-heart surgery is well established [82, 83]. Some studies have shown

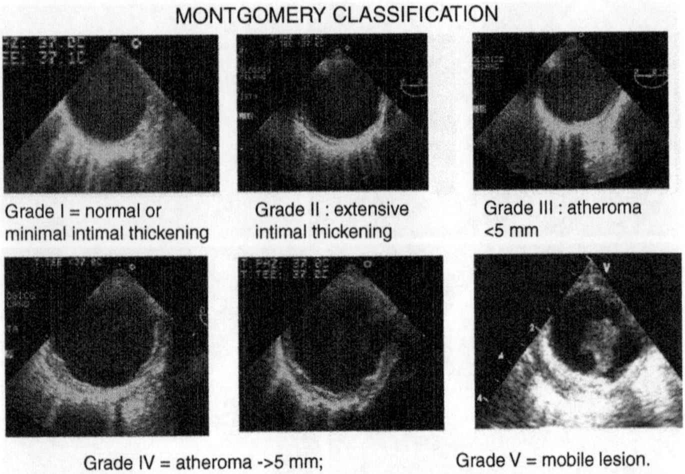

MONTGOMERY CLASSIFICATION

Grade I = normal or
minimal intimal thickening

Grade II : extensive
intimal thickening

Grade III : atheroma
<5 mm

Grade IV = atheroma ->5 mm;

Grade V = mobile lesion.

FIGURE 1.5 Grading system for severity of atherosclerosis in the thoracic aorta proposed by Montgomery. Grade I=normal or minimal intimal thickening; Grade II: extensive intimal thickening; Grade III=atheroma <5 mm; Grade IV=atheroma ≥5 mm; Grade V=mobile lesion. All examples refer to short axis of the descending aorta

the risk of stroke or peripheral embolism after cardiac catheterization or intra-aortic balloon pump placement in patients with severe aortic atherosclerosis diagnosed by TEE [82]. A strong association between aortic stenosis and aortic atherosclerosis has recently been established [84]. The presence of plaques in the aorta of patients with aortic stenosis has important implications since these patients often undergo invasive diagnostic and therapeutic procedures that can dislodge particularly thick plaques and the attached thrombotic material. Large mobile aortic thrombi are possible causes of systemic emboli and appear to be a complication of atherosclerosis. TEE is the best technique for diagnosing and monitoring the evolution of these large thrombi [85]. Figure 1.6 shows a three-dimensional image of large complex plaques in the thoracic aorta of a patient undergoing TAVI for severe aortic stenosis.

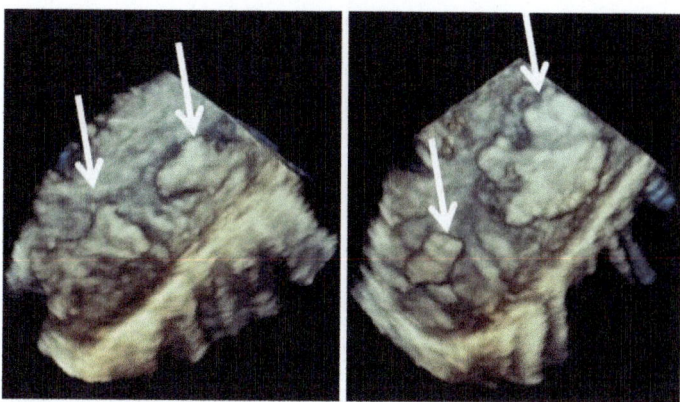

FIGURE 1.6 3D transoesophageal imaging of atheromas of the descending aorta. *Arrows* show several athoromas in two segments of the thoracic descending aorta visualized in a longitudinal view. 3D imaging allows a more detailed view of the complexity of plaques which are irregular in shape and extension

Epiaortic Ultrasonography

In epiaortic imaging, the transducer is placed directly over the aortic arch in a surgical setting. Although it allows us to image aortic arch plaque the information derived is usually used to select operative techniques in order to reduce the risk of perioperative strokes [86, 87].

Magnetic Resonance (MR) Imaging

MR may be used for detection and measurement of aortic arch plaque [77, 88] and to monitor aortic plaque progression and regression [86]. Contrast MR is also used to identify morphological features such as calcification, thrombus, fibrocellular tissue and lipids which may be useful to detect plaque stability.

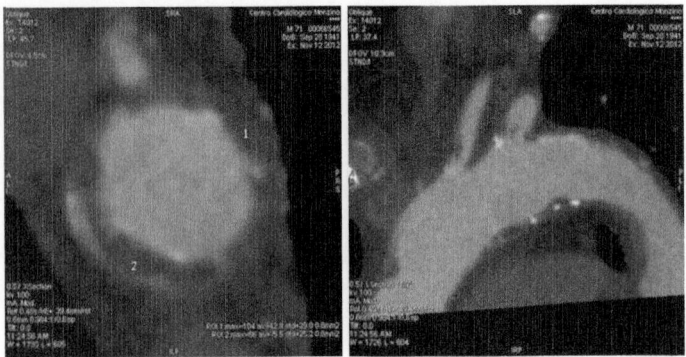

FIGURE 1.7 Atheromas of the aortic arch visualised by cardiac computed tomography; the white small spots visualised in the short (*left*) or long (*right*) images indicated calcified deposition inside the aortic wall, while the small diffused indentation of the walls (black spots) are due to parietal atheromas

Contrast MR angiography may underestimate the plaque thickness and its use may be limited in obese or claustrophobic patients as well as in subjects who have metallic implants.

Computed Tomography (CT)

Multidetector CT has been demonstrated to be an accurate and powerful tool for detecting atheroma in extra- and intracranial vessels. CT is the test of choice for detecting vascular calcification and can reliably detect and measure protruding aortic plaques [77, 89]. CT identifies more plaques throughout the aortic arch and around the origins of the major cerebral arteries in particular compared to TEE (Fig. 1.7). These may represent potential embolic sources of acute ischaemic stroke. Better plaque detection may have an impact on the best available secondary prevention regimen in individual patients if proximal embolic sources are suspected. MDCT allows evaluation of the whole arterial vasculature. In addition, MDCT has the ability to visualize the vessel wall and to give a quantitative measurement of calcified and noncalcified plaque.

However, CT may underestimate the amount of non-calcified plaque and mobile thrombus that presumably is at high risk for embolisation [77]. In conjunction with positron emission tomography, it can be used to localise fluorodeoxyglucose uptake by the plaque, identifying active plaques and plaques prone to rupture (unstable) [90], but its clinical utility has yet to be established.

Concerning specifically pre-operative (cardiac surgery) evaluation, preoperative CT scans in patients at high risk may help identify aortic areas at risk before entering the operating room, lead to more thorough screening in the operating room, and result in a more aggressive strategy to avoid calcified areas.

Microembolic Signals by Transcranial Doppler (TCD) Ultrasonography

The occurrence of microembolic signals, as detected by transcranial Doppler (TCD) ultrasonography, can be a marker of severe aortic atherosclerosis, and monitoring these signals should enable the application of appropriate surgical methods to coronary artery bypass patients who are at higher risk of stroke [91]. Asymptomatic cerebral embolic signals (ES) may be associated with severe (≥4 mm) aortic arch atherosclerosis but not with aortic arch atherosclerosis <4 mm or no aortic arch atherosclerosis [92].

Contrast Aortography

The need for contrast injection and radiation as well as the risk of iatrogenic complications due to the invasive nature of the procedure make this technique rarely used to assess aortic plaques [93].

Treatment of Aortic Atheroma

There are no published and conclusive randomised trials to guide the therapy of aortic embolism. So, only strategies for general atherosclerosis management are usually recommended.

Beside nonspecific risk modification (e.g. smoking cessation), strategies include medical, surgical, and interventional therapy.

Medical Therapy

Treatment of Aortic Atheroma Without Embolic Events

As both types of aortic embolisms (thromboembolism and atheroembolism) occur more frequently in the context of atherosclerosis, strategies devoted to the control of atherosclerosis risk factors, including smoking cessation and pharmacological control of conventional risk factors such as blood pressure, lipids and diabetes, may indirectly prevent the embolism from aortic plaques. Even if ad hoc clinical trials are needed to determine the effects of anti–atherosclerotic and antiplatelet treatments in patients with severe aortic atheroma and risk of atheroembolism, on the basis of general guidelines for primary and secondary prevention of atherosclerosis–related events, proposed pharmacological therapies for aortic embolism include statins and antiplatelet agents.

Statins

A body of indirect evidence, obtained in a variety of patient cohorts, suggests that statins may reduce the risk of stroke [4, 94]. For example, in an observational study of 519 patients with severe aortic plaques documented by TEE, statin use resulted in a relative risk reduction for ischaemic stroke of 59 % [64].

Plaque regression in the thoracic aorta and retardation of plaque progression in the abdominal aorta by 1-year atorvastatin (20 mg versus 5 mg) have also been reported in an MRI prospective, randomised, open–label trial carried out in 36 hypercholesterolaemic patients [95]. After 2 years of treatment, regression of thoracic plaques was found in the 20 mg group (−15 % vessel wall area reduction), but not in the 5 mg group (+7 %). Regarding abdominal plaques, progression was found in the 5 mg group (+10 %), but not in the 20 mg group (+2 %). The degree of thoracic plaque regression correlated with LDL–cholesterol reduction (r = 0.61), whereas thoracic plaque change from 1 to 2 years correlated with on–treatment LDL–cholesterol levels (r = 0.64). In the abdominal aorta, only retardation of plaque progression was found after 2 years of 20 mg treatment [95].

The incidence of stroke may be reduced by statins not only through their conventional lipid-lowering effect, but also with other mechanisms; the so called "pleiotropic effects", which include plaque regression/stabilisation, reduction in the inflammatory response, and inhibition of the coagulation cascade at different levels. For example, a regression of thoracic aortic plaques after lipid–lowering therapy with simvastatin was demonstrated using MRI [96, 97]. Other two MRI randomized studies evaluated the effects of aggressive vs conventional lipid-lowering therapy in patients with aortic and/or carotid plaques and reported significant plaque regression which was significantly associated with the reduction in LDL cholesterol [98, 99]. In one of the two studies, a relationship with the statin dosage was also observed [99].

On these bases, despite the lack of *ad hoc* randomized trials, there are guidelines clearly stating that: "*a treatment with a statin is a reasonable option for patients with aortic arch atheroma to reduce the risk of stroke*" [8] (Table 1.2). In addition, it has to be kept in mind that statins are recommended for many manifestations of atherosclerotic diseases; therefore, a large number of patients with identified aortic plaque already have indications for statins for secondary prevention for cerebrovascular diseases [100].

Anticoagulation Versus Antiplatelet Therapy

Coexistent severe aortic atherosclerosis could affect prothrombotic profiles of patients with atrial fibrillation (AF). Being at risk for thromboembolism, such patients seem to have an indication for an intensive antithrombotic therapy

TABLE 1.2 Treatment recommendations for uncomplicated aortic atheroma, complicated atheroma, suspected aortic embolic event, large thrombi

Therapy	Recommendations	Class[a]	Level[b]
Uncomplicated atheroma			
Statin is a reasonable option for patients with aortic arch atheroma to reduce the risk of stroke	Recommended [8]	IIa	C
Oral anticoagulation therapy with warfarin (INR 2.0–3.0) or antiplatelet therapy	Reasonable in stroke patients with aortic arch atheroma 4.0 mm or greater to prevent recurrent stroke [8]	IIb	C
Patients with thoracic aortic atheroma, not requiring surgery, as well as for patients who are not considered to be surgical or stent graft candidates			
Stringent control of hypertension	Recommended [8, 100]	I	B/C
Lipid profile optimization	Recommended [8]	IIA	A
Smoking cessation, and other atherosclerosis risk-reduction measures	Recommended [8]	I	B
Patients with thoracic aortic atheroma undergoing cardiac surgical procedures requiring cardiopulmonary bypass (coronary bypass surgery and valve surgery)			
Endarterectomy of aortic arch plaque for the purposes of secondary stroke prevention	not recommended [101]		

Complicated aortic atheroma and/or suspected aortic embolic event and/or Large aortic thrombi

Patients with an ischemic stroke or TIA and evidence of aortic arch atheroma

		Class of evidence[a]	Level of certainty[b]
Antiplatelet therapy	Recommended [102]	I	A
Statin therapy	Recommended [102, 103]	I	A [103], B [102]
Anticoagulation with warfarin	Effectiveness unknown [102]	IIB	C
Endarterectomy of aortic arch plaque for the purposes of secondary stroke prevention	not recommended [102]	III	C

Patients with native aortic disease who do not have AF or another indication for anticoagulation

Antiplatelet therapy	Recommended [102]	I	C

[a]Class of evidence
[b]Level of certainty

[104]. Patients with nonrheumatic AF who have spontaneous echocardiographic contrast in the descending thoracic aorta appear to have enhanced coagulation activity but not platelet activity [105]. Cholesterol emboli on skin, muscle, and renal biopsy samples often occur in patients with aortic arch atheroma [42], but there is also evidence, even if coming from small scale studies, which shows that the prevalence of clinical atheroemboli syndrome is lower when patients are treated with warfarin, thus suggesting a potential benefit of this therapy in patients with aortic arch atheroma.

A second observational TEE study [106] was carried out in 129 patients with aortic arch atheroma to investigate the source of cerebral or peripheral embolisation. In this non-randomised study, the antithrombotic therapy (oral anticoagulation, aspirin, or ticlopidine) was left to the discretion of the practitioner in charge of the patient. At the end of follow-up (22 ± 10 months), a significant reduction in the number of embolic events among patients who received oral anticoagulants (0 events in 27 patients versus 5 events in 23 patients treated with antiplatelet agents) was noted even if just in patients with plaques $\geq$ to 4 mm.

The SPAF (Stroke Prevention in Atrial Fibrillation) trial [61] was a randomised study carried out to define TEE predictors of stroke in patients with atrial fibrillation and to examine response to antithrombotic therapy. A total of 382 patients with atrial fibrillation at high risk for thromboembolism have been included into the study. Among patients with "high–risk" non–valvular atrial fibrillation, the 1-year risk of stroke in 134 patients with complex aortic plaque was found to be reduced from 15.8 % (11 events) in those treated with fixed low–dose warfarin plus aspirin (INR 1.2–1.5) to 4 % (3 events) in those treated with adjusted–dose warfarin (INR 2.0–3.0), which means a 75 % relative risk reduction ($P = 0.02$) for patients with atheromas who received "therapeutic range" anticoagulation [61].

All these reports suggest that warfarin in patients with aortic arch atheroma is not harmful and may reduce the rate of stroke. Therefore, intensive anticoagulation treatment seems to be a reasonable option for patients with aortic atheroma and the 2010 ACCF/AHA/AATS/ACR/ASA/SCA/SCAI/SIR/STS/SVM Guidelines [8] suggest that oral anticoagulation therapy with warfarin (INR 2.0–3.0) or antiplatelet therapy may be considered in stroke patients with aortic arch atheroma 4.0 mm or greater to prevent recurrent stroke.

Despite these indications, the use of anticoagulation in patients with aortic plaques, even in those with thrombogenic mobile components, is still controversial. Indeed, retrospective information show no significant benefit of warfarin or antiplatelet drugs on the incidence of stroke and other embolic events in patients with severe thoracic aortic plaques on TEE [64]. In addition, in other small scale studies, either harmful or beneficial effects of anticoagulation were reported and anticoagulation has been associated with both worsening [21, 107], and improvement of an aortic thrombus in a patient with the atheroemboli syndrome [108]. Moreover, the use of warfarin in patients with aortic atheroma may be harmful also because of the theoretical risk of plaque haemorrhage, which may result in atheroemboli syndrome (i.e. blue toes, renal failure and intestinal infarction) [109].

It has to be underlined that all the studies published so far were not randomised trials and that they are not specifically designed for treatment of patients with aorta atheromas, and that the sample size is always relatively small. So, the ideal therapeutic approach to these patients still awaits prospective randomized double blind evaluation.

As for statins, it has to be underlined, however, that many patients with aortic embolism already have a strong indication for the use of antiplatelet agents for secondary prevention of cardio- and cerebrovascular events.

Thrombolytic Agents

In acute cerebral thromboembolism, thrombolytic agents may be used to restore blood flow in the affected vessel. There is evidence showing that mobile aortic atheroma may disappear with the use of these drugs [110].

Treatment of Aortic Atheroma After Stroke or Suspected Embolic Event

Statins

Despite the absence of randomized clinical trials specifically designed to evaluate the effectiveness of statin therapy for reducing the risk of recurrent stroke among patients with complex aortic plaque, observational studies in patients with a recent embolic event, including stroke or TIA, suggest that this class of drugs may be effective in preventing recurrent events [64]. On these basis, recent guidelines [102, 103] recommend statins to reduce the risk of stroke and cardiovascular events among patients with ischemic stroke or TIA who have evidence of aortic atherosclerosis (Table 1.2).

Anticoagulation Versus Antiplatelet Therapy

Data on the use of anticoagulant or antiplatelet therapy for secondary prevention of atheroembolism are quite inconsistent. As for statins, also in this case randomized clinical trials are lacking, and the observational studies available are small and results mixed [25, 81, 106, 111].

The ARCH (Aortic Arch Related Cerebral Hazard) trial is the unique open–label trial testing the usefulness of full–dose anticoagulation with warfarin (target INR 2.0–3.0) against a combination of low–dose aspirin (75 mg/day) plus clopidogrel (75 mg/day) for prevention of recurrent vascular events in patients with aortic atheroma (4 mm or greater) and non–disabling stroke [112]. Unfortunately, although completed, the results of this study have not yet been published (Table 1.2).

Endarterectomy or Cover Stents

In a study designed to assess the risks or benefits of aortic arch endarterectomy for reducing the risk of recurrent aortic atheroembolism and intraoperative stroke during cardiac surgery provided unpromising results [14]. Arch endarterectomy was performed in 43 of 268 patients who had arch atheromas ≥5 mm or with mobile components on intraoperative TEE [14]. The overall mortality and the incidence of intraoperative stroke were rather high (14.9 % and 15.3 %, respectively) and, on multivariate analysis, aortic arch endarterectomy was even an independent predictor of intraoperative stroke (OR, 3.6; P=0.001). A possible alternative to endarterectomy to prevent embolization might be the use of cover stents, which may have the potential advantage of shielding severely diseased aortic segments. Unfortunately, interventional endovascular manipulations or diagnosis may induce periprocedural embolization. As a consequence also in this case there is no sufficient evidence to recommend prophylactic endarterectomy or aortic arch stenting for purposes of stroke prevention, and therefore surgical guidelines for the management of thoracic aortic disease do not recommend prophylactic endarterectomy or aortic arch stenting for purposes of stroke prevention [101] (Table 1.2).

Treatment of Large Aortic Thrombi

Large Mobile Aortic Thrombi

Mobile thoracic or abdominal thrombi in a nonaneurysmal, minimally atherosclerotic or normal aorta is a rare clinical entity and an uncommon cause of embolism to visceral organs or lower limbs [113–117]. These may be the consequence of underlying pathology such as hypercoagulable disorders [113, 118, 119], concurrent malignancy [113], periprocedural outcomes [120], anticancer treatments e.g. cisplatin-based chemotherapy [121], Crohn's Disease [122], protein C deficiency [123], essential thrombocytosis [124], and traumatic aortic injury [125]. The discovery of an aortic thrombus may be even incidental [126].

Because of the rarity of this condition there is a paucity of case reports. Both anticoagulation therapy and aortic surgery or both [127, 128], are commonly used as primary treatment, but there are no consensuses or clinical guidelines to outline the best management strategy for this unusual problem. No long-term follow up of this rare pathology is available.

According to a number of case report studies endovascular stent graft placement is feasible and can be performed as an effective and minimally invasive treatment option for mobile thoracic aortic thrombi [129–137]. Surgical removal of the aortic thrombus may be another options [114, 117, 123, 138–144].

Treatment strategy for thrombus originating from an almost normal thoracic aorta remains controversial [145]. According to some authors, the indication for surgical intervention results from contraindication to anticoagulation, mobile thrombus or recurrent embolism. Whenever possible, endovascular therapy should be preferred [113].

Anticoagulants

In studies carried out in patients with aortic mobile lesions documented by TEE [25, 146], the authors described an incidence of vascular events much lower in patients treated with warfarin than in those who were not treated (5 % versus 45 %). In addition, mobile aortic atheromas have been noted to disappear during anticoagulant therapy, in some [34, 108, 147], but not all studies [148]. In the SPAF trial [61] the trend toward fewer embolic events while on anticoagulants in patients with mobile lesions, did not reach statistical significance, whereas the mortality was significantly reduced [61].

A systematic review including a meta-analysis including 98 articles compares the outcomes of anticoagulation therapy and aortic surgery strategies for the treatment of aortic mural thrombus. Two hundred patients were considered: 112 received anticoagulation and 88 underwent aortic surgery as primary treatment. The results of the meta-analysis seem to favor the surgical management of aortic mural thrombus in the normal or minimally diseased aorta. Indeed, although mortality rates were similar (6.2 % and 5.7 % for the anticoagulation group and the surgery group, respectively; P = 0.879), anticoagulation as primary therapy was associated with a higher likelihood of recurrence of peripheral arterial embolization (25.7 % Vs. 9.1 %; P = 0.003), a trend toward a higher incidence of complications (27 % Vs. 17 %; P = 0.07), a higher likelihood of major limb amputation (9 % Vs. 2 %; P = 0.004). In addition, aortic thrombus persisted or recurred in 26.4 % of the anticoagulation group and in 5.7 % of the surgery group (P < 0.001). Multivariable logistic analysis established thrombus location in the ascending aorta or arch, mild atherosclerosis of the aortic wall and stroke presentation as important predictors of recurrence. On these basis the authors concluded that aortic surgery should be considered as primary treatment, particularly for those patients at high risk for recurrence considered to be good operative candidates [149].

Thrombolysis

Some case report studies suggest thrombolysis as another possible strategy to treat aortic thrombi [150, 151].

In conclusion in the literature there is no consensus how to treat a symptomatic floating aortic thrombus. This report shows that therapeutic strategies are influenced by the localisation of the thrombus, the co-morbidities of the patient and the physician' s preferences. Endovascular *treatment* in combination with high dose statins has become the preferred *treatment* although long-term data are lacking [115].

Large Fix Aortic Thrombi

To date, there are no evidence-based data to support specific drug therapy for a patient with atheroembolism and large fix or mobile aortic thrombi. It makes sense to use statins in any patient with atherosclerosis, as these drugs have been shown to reduce the risk of myocardial infarction and stroke, and have a theoretical benefit on plaque stabilization. Surgical treatment should be considered for patients with abdominal aortic or popliteal artery aneurysms and downstream atheroembolism.

There are case reports of atheroemboli in patients worsening after given warfarin or heparin. For this reason, some institutions are reluctant to prescribe these drugs for patients with atheroemboli or thromboemboli from aortic plaque. However, the incidence of this complication is quite low. Similarly, the current state of knowledge does not allow for selecting specific pharmacologic intervention in patients with thromboemboli from fix aortic plaque. Statin therapy does make sense, as these drugs theoretically stabilize plaques and prevent plaque hemorrhage, thrombosis, and subsequent embolization. Unstable aortic plaques may develop superimposed thrombi (red thrombi on pathologic examination), easily seen as mobile elements on TEE. Therefore, it is possible that anticoagulation with warfarin might prevent embolic events in these patients. For this reason, we are often in the position of recommending warfarin therapy for patients with emboli and severe atheromas seen on TEE, especially when superimposed mobile thrombi are seen. There are small series in the literature that indicate the potential benefit of warfarin.

Large fix aortic thrombi are a very common finding particularly in old patients with conventional and non conventional atherosclerotic risk factor. As previously underlined plaque thickness of ≥4 mm is associated with a significantly increased embolic risk. In an MRI study in aortic and carotid lesions on the effects of aggressive versus conventional lipid lowering therapy by simvastatin, treatment was associated with a significant regression of atherosclerotic lesions. Plaque regression was more related to the degree of LDL-C reduction rather than to the dose of statin, because no difference between high- and moderate dose simvastatin was detected.

Surgical and Interventional Therapy

In acute aortic thromboembolism, interventional approaches may be used to treat end–organ ischaemia (e.g. percutaneous intervention to restore the flow of a cerebral artery occluded by a thromboembolus). Covered stents, endarterectomy and even arterial bypass surgery have been used in a small number of patients with aortic embolism with limited success. Some authors suggest that mural aortic thrombi can be successfully treated with a definitive surgical procedure in selected patients, with low mortality and morbidity [57]. Despite this, at the moment there is no convincing evidence to recommend either endarterectomy or aortic stenting for stroke prevention in patients with thoracic aortic plaques [8]. Indeed, although a handful of case reports on aortic arch endarterectomy in patients with thromboembolism originating from aortic arch atheroma have reported successful results, this procedure seems to be associated with a relatively high rate of perioperative stroke and mortality (34.9 % with endarterectomy versus 11.6 % without endarterectomy), especially when performed to limit stroke during cardiac surgical procedures requiring cardiopulmonary bypass (coronary bypass surgery and valve surgery) [14]. Even if covered stents may offer the potential advantage of shielding severely diseased aortic segments to prevent further embolisation, peri–procedural embolisation may occur during diagnosis or interventional endovascular manipulations. Endovascular stenting for treatment of aortic embolism has largely been limited to abdominal aortic and infrainguinal forms of the disease [134].

Randomised blinded controlled trials are therefore needed to test currently available treatment options, both medical and surgical, to prevent embolic vascular events.

Follow-up of Aortic Atherosclerosis or Large Thrombi

No data exist in this filed. Large fix aortic plaques are a very common finding particularly in old patients with conventional and non conventional atherosclerotic risk factor and are associated in several cases to stratified thrombi. As previously underlined plaque thickness of ≥ 4 mm is associated with a significantly increased embolic risk. Therefore an aggressive treatment with anticoagulant plus statins may be reasonably advocated even though data on this topic are lacking.

DRUG Interactions

As stated before, proposed pharmacological therapies for aortic atheroma include mainly statins, anticoagulation and antiplatelet agents. To use these drugs in the most effective and safest manner, it could be useful for clinicians to have an understanding of mechanisms of potential drug interactions, which drug interactions have already been described and which drug interactions may at least theoretically occur. Since it would be impossible to describe all potential interactions, only those potentially occurring among statins, anticoagulants and antiplatelet agents will be described.

Interactions Affecting Lipid-Lowering Drugs

Although generally well tolerated, lipid–lowering drugs may be involved in different types of drug–drug interactions [152, 153], which generally fall under two categories: pharmacokinetic (i.e. how the body processes the drug) and pharmacodynamic (i.e. how the drug affects the body).

Interactions Affecting Statins

Statin interactions may have either a pharmacokinetic or pharmacodynamic basis, or both (Table 1.3) and it is now widely accepted that knowledge of the pharmacokinetic and pharmacodynamic properties of statins should avoid the majority of drug interactions. Pharmacokinetic interactions may be associated with adverse events such as myopathy and rhabdomyolysis, and to either an enhanced or reduced lipid lowering effect. Pharmacokinetic interactions may take place at any stage of absorption, distribution, metabolism, or excretion. An important role in statin metabolism is played by the cytochrome P450 (CYP) enzyme system; however, a level of difficulty in predicting possible statin interactions lies in the fact that different statins are metabolised by different CYP enzymes and to

TABLE 1.3 Effects of co-prescribed drugs interfering with the absorption, metabolism or pharmacodynamic of statins

Co-prescribed treatment	Statin	Possible effects
Interference with absorption		
Bile–acid sequestrants	Pravastatin [154] Simvastatin [155] Fluvastatin [156]	Absorption reduction
Dietary fibre	Lovastatin [157]	Absorption reduction
Oral antacid containing magnesium and aluminium hydroxides	Rosuvastatin [158]	Plasma concentration reduced
Reduction of gastric acidity with H$_2$-receptor antagonist (Cimetidine, ranitidine) Proton pump inhibitor (omeprazole)	Fluvastatin [152]	Increase plasma concentration without major clinical significance [156, 159, 160]
Food	Pravastatin [161] Fluvastatin [156, 162] Atorvastatin [163]	Systemic bioavailability reduced (poor clinical significance)
Food	Lovastatin [164]	Absorption increased (poor clinical significance)
Herbal medicines (St. John's wort)	Simvastatin [165]	Plasma concentration reduced

(continued)

TABLE 1.3 (continued)

Co-prescribed treatment	Statin	Possible effects
Herbal medicines (wheat bran)	Lovastatin [165]	Plasma concentration reduced
P-glycoprotein inhibitors	Statins [166]	Influence on oral bioavailability
Aspirin	Statins [167]	No pharmacokinetic interactions
Dual antiplatelet therapy (aspirin and clopidogrel)	Atorvastatin or fluvastatin [168, 169]	No pharmacokinetic interactions
Ticagrelor	Atorvastatin and simvastatin [170, 171]	Statin plasma concentration modestly augmented (atorvastatin) or larger augmented (simvastatin)
Interference with the metabolism		
CYP3A4 inhibitors (e.g. cyclosporin)	Statins [166]	Increased statin exposure possibly leading to myopathy and rhabdomyolysis
Itraconazole	Simvastatin [172] Statins [173]	Increased statin exposure possibly leading to myopathy and rhabdomyolysis
Azole antifungals, macrolides, azalides, HIV protease inhibitors	Statins [152, 174, 175]	Clinically significant interactions may occur

Pharmacodynamic interactions (may lead to either synergism or antagonism)

Gemfibrozil	Cerivastatin [166]	Rhabdomyolysis
Aspirin	Statins [176]	Positive interaction: additive effect in reducing cardiovascular events
Thienopyridines (ticlopidine and clopidogrel)	Statins [177, 178]	Recommendation in [179]
Clopidogrel	Statins [180–193]	No relevant interactions
Clopidogrel	Lipophilic statins [179, 192, 194, 195]	Diminished anti platelet activity of clopidogrel
Prasugrel	Statins [196, 197]	No relevant interactions

Statins may inhibit platelets directly with yet unidentified mechanism(s) perhaps related to the regulation of the PAR–1 thrombin receptors [187] different degrees and in some cases the metabolism produces active metabolites. Lovastatin, simvastatin and atorvastatin are metabolised by the CYP3A family. Fluvastatin is metabolised by CYP2C9 whereas pravastatin is not significantly metabolised by the CYP system [166]. If concurrent therapy with known inhibitors of statin metabolism is needed, patients should be monitored for signs and symptoms of myopathy or rhabdomyolysis possibly reducing the dosage or even discontinuing the statin therapy if needed [166].

Of course, statins may also affect the metabolism and consequent concentrations of other coadministered therapies, such as digoxin, leading to alterations in effect or a requirement for clinical monitoring.

Warfarin Drug–Drug Interactions

Warfarin can interact, at least potentially, with a large number of drugs by both pharmacokinetic and pharmacodynamic mechanisms (Table 1.4). Warfarin is a racemic mixture of S and R isomers. The two isomers are metabolized by two different cytochrome P450 enzymes: CYP2C9 (which metabolizes the S isomer) and CYP3A4 (which metabolizes R isomer). As the S isomer is five times more potent than the R isomer, drug interactions involving the S isomer have usually a higher clinical importance. Knowledge on whether co–prescribed drugs are metabolized by these two CYP enzymes allows a reasonable INR change prediction and possible subsequent bleeding (Tables 1.5 and 1.6).

TABLE 1.4 Effects of co-prescribed drugs interfering with the metabolism or the clearance of warfarin

Mechanism	Examples	Possible effects
CYP2C9 induction	Rifampicin [198, 199]	INR reduction
CYP2C9 inhibition	Fluconazole [198–200] Fluvoxamine [198, 201]	strong INR increase
CYP3A4 induction	St John's wort [202]	INR reduction
CYP3A4 inhibition	Clarithromycin [199] Fluconazole [198, 199] Simvastatin [199, 203]	INR increase
Interference with the clearance of warfarin	Underlying condition for which the antibiotic is prescribed (eg. Pneumonia) [204] Antibiotics [205, 206]	INR increase
Interference with clearance of the R isomer of warfarin	Diltiazem [207] Antibiotics [208, 209]	Modest INR increase
Interference with the clearance of both warfarin isomers	Amiodarone [210, 211]	Strong INR increase
Interference with the amount of vitamin K produced by the intestinal bacteria	Antibiotics [204, 206]	INR increase
Reduction of vitamin K intake	Dietary changes associated to antibiotics treatments [204]	INR increase

TABLE 1.5 Examples of substrates, inhibitors, and inducers of CYP2C9

Substrates	Inhibitors	Inducers
NSAIDs (analgesic, antipyretic, anti–inflammatory): Celecoxib [212] Lornoxicam [213] Diclofenac [212] Ibuprofen [212] Naproxen [212] Piroxicam [212] Meloxicam [213] Suprofen [212] Flurbiprofen [212] Mefenamic acid [212]	**Strong:** Antifungal azoles: Fluconazole [214] Miconazole [214] Voriconazole [214]	**Strong:** Rifampicin [214] (bactericidal) Dexamethasone [214] (Glucocorticoid) Bosentan [214] (endothelin receptor antagonist)
	Valproic acid [214] (Anticonvulsant)	Phenobarbital [214] (Barbiturate)
	Sulfamethoxazole [214] (Antibacterial) Imatinib [214] (tyrosine–kinase inhibitor)	Anticonvulsants, mood stabilizers: Carbamazepine [214] Phenytoin [214]
	Gemfibrozil [214] (fibrate)	**Unspecified potency:**
	Zafirlukast [214] (leukotriene antagonist)	St. John's Wort [215]
Fluvastatin [212] (Statin)	Amiodarone [214] (Antiarrhythmic)	Secobarbital [216] (Barbiturate)
Ketamine [217] (Sedative)	Fluvastatin [214] (Statin)	
Terbinafine [214] (Antifungal)	**Weak:**	

TABLE 1.5 (continued)

Substrates	Inhibitors	Inducers
Angiotensin II receptor antagonists (in hypertension, diabetic nephropathy, CHF):	Clopidogrel [214] (antiplatelet agent)	
Irbesartan [212]	Curcuma [214]	
Losartan [212]	Irbesartan [214] (Angiotensin II receptor antagonist)	
Sulfonylureas (antidiabetics): Glipizide [212] Glimepiride [212] Tolbutamide [212] Glyburide [212] (or glibenclamide)	Fluvoxamine [214] (Selective serotonin re–uptake inhibitors or SSRI) **Unspecified potency**: Amentoflavone [218] (constituent of Ginkgo biloba and St. John's Wort)	
Other antidiabetics:	Phenylbutazone [219] (NSAID)	
Nateglinide [214]	Flavones or flavonols: [220]	
Rosiglitazone [212]	Quercetin [220]	
S–warfarin [212] (Anticoagulant)	Luteolin [220]	
Phenytoin [212] (Antiepileptic)	Baicalein [220]	
Cyclophosphamide [212] (Alkylating agent)	Wogonin [220] Apigenin [220]	

(continued)

TABLE 1.5 (continued)

Substrates	Inhibitors	Inducers
Sildenafil [212] (in erectile dysfunction)	Sulfaphenazole [216] (Antibacterial)	
Torasemide [212] (Loop diuretic)	H1–receptor antagonists (Antihistamines):	
Amitriptyline [214] (Tricyclic antidepressant)	Cyclizine [221]	
Fluoxetine [212] (SSRI antidepressant)	Promethazine [221]	
Tamoxifen [212] (Selective estrogen–receptor modulator or SERM)	Sertraline [216] (Selective serotonin re–uptake inhibitors or SSRI)	
	Isoniazid [216] (in tuberculosis)	
Others... [212]	Others... [214]	

TABLE 1.6 Examples of substrates, inhibitors, and inducers of CYP3A4

Substrates	Inhibitors	Inducers
	Strong:	Strong:
Statins:	Antifungal azoles:	Anticonvulsants, mood stabilizers
Lovastatin [222]	Itraconazole [222]	Carbamazepine [222]
Simvastatin [222]	Ketoconazole [222]	Phenytoin [222]
Atorvastatin [222]	Miconazole [222]	Barbiturates
Cerivastatin [222] (also metabolised by CYP2C8)	Fluconazole [222]	Phenobarbital [222]
	Voriconazole [222]	Pentobarbital [222]

TABLE 1.5 (continued)

Substrates	Inhibitors	Inducers
Omeprazole [222] (proton pump inhibitor)	Telithromycin [222] (Macrolide antibiotic)	Efavirenz [222] (Non–nucleoside reverse transcriptase inhibitor)

Calcium channel blockers:
    Felodipine [222]
    Nifedipine [222]
    Amlodipine [222]
    Nitrendipine [222]
    Verapamil [222]
    Nisoldipine [222]
    Diltiazem [222]
	Cimetidine [222] (H2–receptor antagonist)
	
	HIV protease inhibitors:
	    Indinavir [214]
	    Ritonavir [214]
	    Nelfinavir [214]
		Dexamethasone [222] (glucocorticoid)
		
		Rifampicin [214] (antibiotic)
		
		Weak:
		
		Steroids:
		    Estradiol [222]
		    Estrogens [222]

	Nefazodone [214] (antidepressant)	Ethanol [214, 223]
R–Warfarin [222] (anticoagulant)	Aprepitant [222] (antiemetic)	Troglitazone [222] (antidiabetic)

Some glucocorticoids:
 	
    Budesonide [222]
 	
    Dexamethasone [222]
	Calcium channel blockers:
	
	    Verapamil [214]
	
	    Diltiazem [214]
		Pantoprazole [222] (proton pump inhibitor)

Clopidogrel, [222] becoming bioactivated (antiplatelet)	Nifedipine [222] (Calcium channel blocker)	Hydrocortisone [222] (glucocorticoid)
Nateglinide [222] (antidiabetic)	Amiodarone [214] (antiarrhythmic)	**Unspecified potency**:
Cyclosporine [222] (inhibitor of calcineurin)	Macrolides antibiotics:	Cigarette smoke [224]

(continued)

TABLE 1.6 (continued)

Substrates	Inhibitors	Inducers
Quinidine [222] (antiarrhythmic)	Erythromycin [214]	Dichlorodiphenyl-trichloroethane (DDT) [225]
	Clarithromycin [214]	
Sildenafil [222] (PDE5 inhibitor)	**Weak**:	Tetrachlorodibenzo –p–dioxin [224]
Benzodiazepines: Alprazolam [222] Midazolam [222] Triazolam [222] Diazepam [222]	Saquinavir [214] (HIV protease inhibitor)	Polycyclic aromatic hydrocarbons [224]
	Chloramphenicol [222] (bacteriostatic antimicrobial)	
	Ciprofloxacin [222] (Antibiotic)	
Finasteride [222] (antiandrogen)	Fluoxetine [214] (Selective serotonin re–uptake inhibitor)	
Estradiol [222] (estrogen)	Lansporazol [222] (proton pump inhibitor)	
Testosterone [222] (androgen)		
Cilostazol [222] (phosphodiesterase inhibitor)	Buprenorphine [222] (analgesic)	
Selective serotonin re–uptake inhibitors (SSRI): Citalopram [222] Sertraline [222]	Valerian [199] Grapefruit juice [199]	
Many others... [222]	Many others... [222]	

References

1. Ferro JM. Cardioembolic stroke: an update. Lancet Neurol. 2003;2(3):177–88. doi:S1474442203003247 [pii].
2. Brickner ME. Cardioembolic stroke. Am J Med. 1996;100(4):465–74. doi:S0002934397895253 [pii].
3. Goldstein LB, Adams R, Alberts MJ, Appel LJ, Brass LM, Bushnell CD, Culebras A, Degraba TJ, Gorelick PB, Guyton JR, Hart RG, Howard G, Kelly-Hayes M, Nixon JV, Sacco RL. Primary prevention of ischemic stroke: a guideline from the American Heart Association/American Stroke Association Stroke Council: cosponsored by the Atherosclerotic Peripheral Vascular Disease Interdisciplinary Working Group; Cardiovascular Nursing Council; Clinical Cardiology Council; Nutrition, Physical Activity, and Metabolism Council; and the Quality of Care and Outcomes Research Interdisciplinary Working Group: the American Academy of Neurology affirms the value of this guideline. Stroke. 2006;37(6):1583–633. doi:10.1161/01.STR.0000223048.70103.F1. 01.STR.0000223048.70103.F1 [pii].
4. Sacco RL, Adams R, Albers G, Alberts MJ, Benavente O, Furie K, Goldstein LB, Gorelick P, Halperin J, Harbaugh R, Johnston SC, Katzan I, Kelly-Hayes M, Kenton EJ, Marks M, Schwamm LH, Tomsick T. Guidelines for prevention of stroke in patients with ischemic stroke or transient ischemic attack: a statement for healthcare professionals from the American Heart Association/American Stroke Association Council on Stroke: co-sponsored by the Council on Cardiovascular Radiology and Intervention: the American Academy of Neurology affirms the value of this guideline. Stroke. 2006;37(2):577–617. doi:10.1161/01.STR.0000199147.30016.74. 37/2/577 [pii].
5. Adams Jr HP, del Zoppo G, Alberts MJ, Bhatt DL, Brass L, Furlan A, Grubb RL, Higashida RT, Jauch EC, Kidwell C, Lyden PD, Morgenstern LB, Qureshi AI, Rosenwasser RH, Scott PA, Wijdicks EF. Guidelines for the early management of adults with ischemic stroke: a guideline from the American Heart Association/American Stroke Association Stroke Council, Clinical Cardiology Council, Cardiovascular Radiology and Intervention Council, and the Atherosclerotic Peripheral Vascular Disease and Quality of Care Outcomes in Research Interdisciplinary Working Groups: the American Academy of Neurology affirms the value of this guideline as an educational tool for neurologists. Stroke. 2007;38(5):1655–711. doi:10.1161/ STROKEAHA.107.181486. STROKEAHA.107.181486 [pii].

6. Flachskampf FA, Badano L, Daniel WG, Feneck RO, Fox KF, Fraser AG, Pasquet A, Pepi M, Perez de Isla L, Zamorano JL, Roelandt JR, Pierard L. Recommendations for transoesophageal echocardiography: update 2010. Eur J Echocardiogr. 2010;11(7):557–76. doi:10.1093/ejechocard/jeq057. jeq057 [pii].

7. Pepi M, Evangelista A, Nihoyannopoulos P, Flachskampf FA, Athanassopoulos G, Colonna P, Habib G, Ringelstein EB, Sicari R, Zamorano JL, Sitges M, Caso P. Recommendations for echocardiography use in the diagnosis and management of cardiac sources of embolism: European Association of Echocardiography (EAE) (a registered branch of the ESC). Eur J Echocardiogr. 2010;11(6):461–76. doi:10.1093/ejechocard/jeq045. jeq045 [pii].

8. Hiratzka LF, Bakris GL, Beckman JA, Bersin RM, Carr VF, Casey Jr DE, Eagle KA, Hermann LK, Isselbacher EM, Kazerooni EA, Kouchoukos NT, Lytle BW, Milewicz DM, Reich DL, Sen S, Shinn JA, Svensson LG, Williams DM. 2010 ACCF/AHA/AATS/ACR/ASA/SCA/SCAI/SIR/STS/SVM Guidelines for the diagnosis and management of patients with thoracic aortic disease. A Report of the American College of Cardiology Foundation/American Heart Association Task Force on Practice Guidelines, American Association for Thoracic Surgery, American College of Radiology, American Stroke Association, Society of Cardiovascular Anesthesiologists, Society for Cardiovascular Angiography and Interventions, Society of Interventional Radiology, Society of Thoracic Surgeons, and Society for Vascular Medicine. J Am Coll Cardiol. 2010;55(14):e27–129. doi:10.1016/j.jacc.2010.02.015.

9. Golledge J, Norman PE. Atherosclerosis and abdominal aortic aneurysm: cause, response, or common risk factors? Arterioscler Thromb Vasc Biol. 2010;30(6):1075–7. doi:10.1161/ATVBAHA.110.206573. 30/6/1075 [pii].

10. Kronzon I, Saric M. Cholesterol embolization syndrome. Circulation. 2010;122(6):631–41. doi:10.1161/CIRCULATIONAHA.109.886465. 122/6/631 [pii].

11. Saric M, Kronzon I. Cholesterol embolization syndrome. Curr Opin Cardiol. 2011;26(6):472–9. doi:10.1097/HCO.0b013e32834b7fdd. 00001573-201111000-00003 [pii].

12. Tunick PA, Kronzon I. Atheromas of the thoracic aorta: clinical and therapeutic update. J Am Coll Cardiol. 2000;35(3):545–54.

13. Tunick PA, Rosenzweig BP, Katz ES, Freedberg RS, Perez JL, Kronzon I. High risk for vascular events in patients with protruding aortic atheromas: a prospective study. J Am Coll Cardiol. 1994;23(5):1085–90.

14. Stern A, Tunick PA, Culliford AT, Lachmann J, Baumann FG, Kanchuger MS, Marschall K, Shah A, Grossi E, Kronzon I. Protruding aortic arch atheromas: risk of stroke during heart surgery with and without aortic arch endarterectomy. Am Heart J. 1999;138(4 Pt 1):746–52.

15. Feder W, Auerbach R. "Purple toes": an uncommon sequela of oral coumarin drug therapy. Ann Intern Med. 1961;55:911–7.

16. Rosansky SJ, Deschamps EG. Multiple cholesterol emboli syndrome after angiography. Am J Med Sci. 1984;288(1):45–8.

17. Hendel RC, Cuenoud HF, Giansiracusa DF, Alpert JS. Multiple cholesterol emboli syndrome. Bowel infarction after retrograde angiography. Arch Intern Med. 1989;149(10):2371–4.

18. Ramirez G, O'Neill Jr WM, Lambert R, Bloomer HA. Cholesterol embolization: a complication of angiography. Arch Intern Med. 1978;138(9):1430–2.

19. Wiseth R, Hallan H, Hatlinghus S, Bjerkeset T, Helseth A. Cholesterol embolization. A serious complication to angiography. Tidsskr Nor Laegeforen. 1988;108(28):2374–6.

20. Drost H, Buis B, Haan D, Hillers JA. Cholesterol embolism as a complication of left heart catheterisation. Report of seven cases. Br Heart J. 1984;52(3):339–42.

21. Hyman BT, Landas SK, Ashman RF, Schelper RL, Robinson RA. Warfarin-related purple toes syndrome and cholesterol microembolization. Am J Med. 1987;82(6):1233–7.

22. Shapiro LS. Cholesterol embolization after treatment with tissue plasminogen activator. N Engl J Med. 1989;321(18):1270. doi:10.1056/NEJM198911023211816.

23. Bols A, Nevelsteen A, Verhaeghe R. Atheromatous embolization precipitated by oral anticoagulants. Int Angiol. 1994;13(3):271–4.

24. Scolari F, Bracchi M, Valzorio B, Movilli E, Costantino E, Savoldi S, Zorat S, Bonardelli S, Tardanico R, Maiorca R. Cholesterol atheromatous embolism: an increasingly recognized cause of acute renal failure. Nephrol Dial Transplant. 1996;11(8):1607–12.

25. Dressler FA, Craig WR, Castello R, Labovitz AJ. Mobile aortic atheroma and systemic emboli: efficacy of anticoagulation and influence of plaque morphology on recurrent stroke. J Am Coll Cardiol. 1998;31(1):134–8. doi:S0735-1097(97)00449-X [pii].

26. Davila-Roman VG, Kouchoukos NT, Schechtman KB, Barzilai B. Atherosclerosis of the ascending aorta is a predictor of renal dysfunction after cardiac operations. J Thorac Cardiovasc Surg. 1999;117(1):111–6. doi:S0022522399000604 [pii].

27. Gutsche JT, Cheung AT, McGarvey ML, Moser WG, Szeto W, Carpenter JP, Fairman RM, Pochettino A, Bavaria JE. Risk factors for perioperative stroke after thoracic endovascular aortic repair. Ann Thorac Surg. 2007;84(4):1195–200; discussion 1200. doi:10.1016/j.athoracsur.2007.04.128. S0003-4975(07)01087-9 [pii].

28. Rodes-Cabau J, Dumont E, Boone RH, Larose E, Bagur R, Gurvitch R, Bedard F, Doyle D, De Larochelliere R, Jayasuria C, Villeneuve J, Marrero A, Cote M, Pibarot P, Webb JG. Cerebral embolism following transcatheter aortic valve implantation: comparison of transfemoral and transapical approaches. J Am Coll Cardiol. 2011;57(1):18–28. doi:10.1016/j. jacc.2010.07.036. S0735-1097(10)04224-5 [pii].

29. Szeto WY, Augoustides JG, Desai ND, Moeller P, McGarvey ML, Walsh E, Bannan A, Herrmann HC, Bavaria JE. Cerebral embolic exposure during transfemoral and transapical transcatheter aortic valve replacement. J Card Surg. 2011;26(4):348–54. doi:10.1111/j.1540-8191.2011.01265.x.

30. Blankenship JC, Butler M, Garbes A. Prospective assessment of cholesterol embolization in patients with acute myocardial infarction treated with thrombolytic vs conservative therapy. Chest. 1995;107(3):662–8.

31. Davila-Roman VG, Barzilai B, Wareing TH, Murphy SF, Schechtman KB, Kouchoukos NT. Atherosclerosis of the ascending aorta. Prevalence and role as an independent predictor of cerebrovascular events in cardiac patients. Stroke. 1994;25(10):2010–6.

32. Amarenco P, Cohen A, Tzourio C, Bertrand B, Hommel M, Besson G, Chauvel C, Touboul PJ, Bousser MG. Atherosclerotic disease of the aortic arch and the risk of ischemic stroke. N Engl J Med.1994;331(22):1474–9.doi:10.1056/NEJM199412013312202.

33. Jones EF, Kalman JM, Calafiore P, Tonkin AM, Donnan GA. Proximal aortic atheroma. An independent risk factor for cerebral ischemia. Stroke. 1995;26(2):218–24.

34. Nihoyannopoulos P, Joshi J, Athanasopoulos G, Oakley CM. Detection of atherosclerotic lesions in the aorta by transesophageal echocardiography. Am J Cardiol. 1993;71(13): 1208–12.

35. Stone DH, Brewster DC, Kwolek CJ, Lamuraglia GM, Conrad MF, Chung TK, Cambria RP. Stent-graft versus open-surgical repair of the thoracic aorta: mid-term results. J Vasc Surg. 2006;44(6):1188–97. doi:10.1016/j.jvs.2006.08.005.

36. Di Tullio MR, Sacco RL, Gersony D, Nayak H, Weslow RG, Kargman DE, Homma S. Aortic atheromas and acute ischemic stroke: a transesophageal echocardiographic study in an ethnically mixed population. Neurology. 1996;46(6):1560–6.

37. Amarenco P, Duyckaerts C, Tzourio C, Henin D, Bousser MG, Hauw JJ. The prevalence of ulcerated plaques in the aortic arch in patients with stroke. N Engl J Med. 1992;326(4):221–5. doi:10.1056/NEJM199201233260402.

38. Khatibzadeh M, Mitusch R, Stierle U, Gromoll B, Sheikhzadeh A. Aortic atherosclerotic plaques as a source of systemic embolism. J Am Coll Cardiol. 1996;27(3):664–9.

39. The French Study of Aortic Plaques in Stroke Group. Atherosclerotic disease of the aortic arch as a risk factor for recurrent ischemic stroke. The French Study of Aortic Plaques in Stroke Group. N Engl J Med. 1996;334(19):1216–21. doi:10.1056/NEJM199605093341902.

40. Di Tullio MR, Sacco RL, Homma S. Atherosclerotic disease of the aortic arch as a risk factor for recurrent ischemic stroke. N Engl J Med. 1996;335(19):1464; author reply 1464–5. doi:10.1056/NEJM199611073351913.

41. Mitusch R, Doherty C, Wucherpfennig H, Memmesheimer C, Tepe C, Stierle U, Kessler C, Sheikhzadeh A. Vascular events during follow-up in patients with aortic arch atherosclerosis. Stroke. 1997;28(1):36–9.

42. Davila-Roman VG, Murphy SF, Nickerson NJ, Kouchoukos NT, Schechtman KB, Barzilai B. Atherosclerosis of the ascending aorta is an independent predictor of long-term neurologic events and mortality. J Am Coll Cardiol. 1999;33(5):1308–16.

43. Cohen A, Tzourio C, Bertrand B, Chauvel C, Bousser MG, Amarenco P. Aortic plaque morphology and vascular events: a follow-up study in patients with ischemic stroke. FAPS Investigators. French Study of Aortic Plaques in Stroke. Circulation. 1997;96(11):3838–41.

44. Sen S, Oppenheimer SM, Lima J, Cohen B. Risk factors for progression of aortic atheroma in stroke and transient ischemic attack patients. Stroke. 2002;33(4):930–5.

45. Montgomery DH, Ververis JJ, McGorisk G, Frohwein S, Martin RP, Taylor WR. Natural history of severe atheromatous disease of the thoracic aorta: a transesophageal echocardiographic study. J Am Coll Cardiol. 1996;27(1):95–101. doi:10.1016/0735-1097(95)00431-9.

46. Pitsavos CE, Aggeli KI, Barbetseas JD, Skoumas IN, Lambrou SG, Frogoudaki AA, Stefanadis CI, Toutouzas PK. Effects of

pravastatin on thoracic aortic atherosclerosis in patients with heterozygous familial hypercholesterolemia. Am J Cardiol. 1998;82(12):1484–8.

47. Geraci A, Weinberger J. Natural history of aortic arch atherosclerotic plaque. Neurology. 2000;54(3):749–51.

48. Sen S, Hinderliter A, Sen PK, Simmons J, Beck J, Offenbacher S, Ohman EM, Oppenheimer SM. Aortic arch atheroma progression and recurrent vascular events in patients with stroke or transient ischemic attack. Circulation. 2007;116(8):928–35. doi:10.1161/CIRCULATIONAHA.106.671727.

49. Blauth CI, Cosgrove DM, Webb BW, Ratliff NB, Boylan M, Piedmonte MR, Lytle BW, Loop FD. Atheroembolism from the ascending aorta. An emerging problem in cardiac surgery. J Thorac Cardiovasc Surg. 1992;103(6):1104–11; discussion 1111–2.

50. Dubrava J, Garay R. The role of transesophageal echocardiography in detection of cardiogenic and aortic sources of embolism in stroke and transient ischaemic attacks. Vnitr Lek. 2006;52(2):144–51.

51. Kessler C, Mitusch R, Guo Y, Rosengart A, Sheikhzadeh A. Embolism from the aortic arch in patients with cerebral ischemia. Thromb Res. 1996;84(3):145–55.

52. Mitusch R, Stierle U, Tepe C, Kummer-Kloess D, Kessler C, Sheikhzadeh A. Systemic embolism in aortic arch atheromatosis. Eur Heart J. 1994;15(10):1373–80.

53. Faggioli GL, Ferri M, Serra C, Biagini E, Manzoli L, Lodi R, Rapezzi C, Stella A. The residual risk of cerebral embolism after carotid stenting: the complex interplay between stent coverage and aortic arch atherosclerosis. Eur J Vasc Endovasc Surg. 2009;37(5):519–24. doi:10.1016/j.ejvs.2008.12.026.

54. Guo Y, Jiang X, Chen S, Zhang S, Zhao H, Wu Y. Aortic arch and intra-/extracranial cerebral arterial atherosclerosis in patients suffering acute ischemic strokes. Chin Med J (Engl). 2003;116(12):1840–4.

55. Tunick PA, Perez JL, Kronzon I. Protruding atheromas in the thoracic aorta and systemic embolization. Ann Intern Med. 1991;115(6):423–7.

56. Shinokawa N, Hirai T, Takashima S, Kameyama T, Nakagawa K, Asanoi H, Inoue H. A transesophageal echocardiographic study on risk factors for stroke in elderly patients with atrial fibrillation: a comparison with younger patients. Chest. 2001;120(3):840–6.

57. Reber PU, Patel AG, Stauffer E, Muller MF, Do DD, Kniemeyer HW. Mural aortic thrombi: an important cause of peripheral embolization. J Vasc Surg. 1999;30(6):1084–9.

58. Harloff A, Simon J, Brendecke S, Assefa D, Helbing T, Frydrychowicz A, Weber J, Olschewski M, Strecker C, Hennig J, Weiller C, Markl M. Complex plaques in the proximal descending aorta: an underestimated embolic source of stroke. Stroke. 2010;41(6):1145–50. doi:10.1161/STROKEAHA.109.577775.

59. Agmon Y, Khandheria BK, Meissner I, Schwartz GL, Petterson TM, O'Fallon WM, Gentile F, Whisnant JP, Wiebers DO, Seward JB. Independent association of high blood pressure and aortic atherosclerosis: a population-based study. Circulation. 2000;102(17):2087–93.

60. Tsimikas S, Brilakis ES, Miller ER, McConnell JP, Lennon RJ, Kornman KS, Witztum JL, Berger PB. Oxidized phospholipids, Lp(a) lipoprotein, and coronary artery disease. N Engl J Med. 2005;353(1):46–57. doi:10.1056/NEJMoa043175. 353/1/46 [pii].

61. Transesophageal echocardiographic correlates of thromboembolism in high-risk patients with nonvalvular atrial fibrillation. The Stroke Prevention in Atrial Fibrillation Investigators Committee on Echocardiography. Ann Intern Med. 1998;128(8):639–47.

62. Agmon Y, Khandheria BK, Meissner I, Petterson TM, O'Fallon WM, Wiebers DO, Christianson TJ, McConnell JP, Whisnant JP, Seward JB, Tajik AJ. C-reactive protein and atherosclerosis of the thoracic aorta: a population-based transesophageal echocardiographic study. Arch Intern Med. 2004;164(16):1781–7. doi:10.1001/archinte.164.16.1781.

63. Konecky N, Malinow MR, Tunick PA, Freedberg RS, Rosenzweig BP, Katz ES, Hess DL, Upson B, Leung B, Perez J, Kronzon I. Correlation between plasma homocyst(e)ine and aortic atherosclerosis. Am Heart J. 1997;133(5):534–40.

64. Tunick PA, Nayar AC, Goodkin GM, Mirchandani S, Francescone S, Rosenzweig BP, Freedberg RS, Katz ES, Applebaum RM, Kronzon I. Effect of treatment on the incidence of stroke and other emboli in 519 patients with severe thoracic aortic plaque. Am J Cardiol. 2002;90(12):1320–5.

65. Tunick PA, Kronzon I. Embolism from the aorta: atheroemboli and thromboemboli. Curr Treat Options Cardiovasc Med. 2001;3(3):181–6.

66. Saric M, Kronzon I. Aortic atherosclerosis and embolic events. Curr Cardiol Rep. 2012;14(3):342–9. doi:10.1007/s11886-012-0261-2.

67. Weinberger J, Azhar S, Danisi F, Hayes R, Goldman M. A new noninvasive technique for imaging atherosclerotic plaque in the aortic arch of stroke patients by transcutaneous real-time B-mode ultrasonography: an initial report. Stroke. 1998; 29(3):673–6.

68. Schwammenthal E, Schwammenthal Y, Tanne D, Tenenbaum A, Garniek A, Motro M, Rabinowitz B, Eldar M, Feinberg MS. Transcutaneous detection of aortic arch atheromas by suprasternal harmonic imaging. J Am Coll Cardiol. 2002;39(7): 1127–32.

69. Tamborini G, Galli CA, Maltagliati A, Andreini D, Pontone G, Quaglia C, Ballerini G, Pepi M. Comparison of feasibility and accuracy of transthoracic echocardiography versus computed tomography in patients with known ascending aortic aneurysm. Am J Cardiol. 2006;98(7):966–9. doi:10.1016/j.amjcard.2006.04.043. S0002-9149(06)01191-X [pii].

70. Mirea O, Maffessanti F, Gripari P, Tamborini G, Muratori M, Fusini L, Claudia C, Fiorentini C, Plesea IE, Pepi M. Effects of aging and body size on proximal and ascending aorta and aortic arch: inner edge-to-inner edge reference values in a large adult population by two-dimensional transthoracic echocardiography. J Am Soc Echocardiogr. 2013;26(4):419–27. doi:10.1016/j. echo.2012.12.013. S0894-7317(12)00982-0 [pii].

71. Kronzon I, Tunick PA. Aortic atherosclerotic disease and stroke. Circulation. 2006;114(1):63–75. doi:10.1161/ CIRCULATIONAHA.105.593418.

72. Katz ES, Konecky N, Tunick PA, Rosenzweig BP, Freedberg RS, Kronzon I. Visualization and identification of the left common carotid and left subclavian arteries: a transesophageal echocardiographic approach. J Am Soc Echocardiogr. 1996;9(1):58–61.

73. Demopoulos LA, Tunick PA, Bernstein NE, Perez JL, Kronzon I. Protruding atheromas of the aortic arch in symptomatic patients with carotid artery disease. Am Heart J. 1995;129(1):40–4. doi:0002-8703(95)90040-3 [pii].

74. Nishino M, Masugata H, Yamada Y, Abe H, Hori M, Kamada T. Evaluation of thoracic aortic atherosclerosis by transesophageal echocardiography. Am Heart J. 1994;127(2):336–44.

75. Vaduganathan P, Ewton A, Nagueh SF, Weilbaecher DG, Safi HJ, Zoghbi WA. Pathologic correlates of aortic plaques, thrombi and mobile "aortic debris" imaged in vivo with transesophageal echocardiography. J Am Coll Cardiol. 1997;30(2):357–63. doi:S0735-1097(97)00181-2 [pii].

76. Laperche T, Laurian C, Roudaut R, Steg PG. Mobile thrombo-ses of the aortic arch without aortic debris. A transesophageal echocardiographic finding associated with unexplained arterial embolism. The Filiale Echocardiographie de la Societe Francaise de Cardiologie. Circulation. 1997;96(1):288–94.

77. Tenenbaum A, Garniek A, Shemesh J, Fisman EZ, Stroh CI, Itzchak Y, Vered Z, Motro M. Dual-helical CT for detecting aortic atheromas as a source of stroke: comparison with trans-esophageal echocardiography. Radiology. 1998;208(1):153–8.

78. Blanchard DG, Kimura BJ, Dittrich HC, DeMaria AN. Transesophageal echocardiography of the aorta. JAMA. 1994; 272(7):546–51.

79. Zaidat OO, Suarez JI, Hedrick D, Redline S, Schluchter M, Landis DM, Hoit B. Reproducibility of transesophageal echo-cardiography in evaluating aortic atheroma in stroke patients. Echocardiography. 2005;22(4):326–30. doi:10.1111/j.1540-8175.2005.04044.x.

80. Meissner I, Khandheria BK, Sheps SG, Schwartz GL, Wiebers DO, Whisnant JP, Covalt JL, Petterson TM, Christianson TJ, Agmon Y. Atherosclerosis of the aorta: risk factor, risk marker, or innocent bystander? A prospective population-based trans-esophageal echocardiography study. J Am Coll Cardiol. 2004;44(5):1018–24. doi:10.1016/j.jacc.2004.05.075.

81. Di Tullio MR, Russo C, Jin Z, Sacco RL, Mohr JP, Homma S. Aortic arch plaques and risk of recurrent stroke and death. Circulation. 2009;119(17):2376–82. doi:10.1161/CIRCULATIONAHA.108.811935. CIRCULATIONAHA.108.811935 [pii].

82. Keeley EC, Grines CL. Scraping of aortic debris by coronary guiding catheters: a prospective evaluation of 1,000 cases. J Am Coll Cardiol. 1998;32(7):1861–5. doi:S0735109798004975 [pii].

83. van der Linden J, Hadjinikolaou L, Bergman P, Lindblom D. Postoperative stroke in cardiac surgery is related to the location and extent of atherosclerotic disease in the ascending aorta. J Am Coll Cardiol. 2001;38(1):131–5. doi:S0735-1097(01)01328-6 [pii].

84. Osranek M, Pilip A, Patel PR, Molisse T, Tunick PA, Kronzon I. Amounts of aortic atherosclerosis in patients with aortic steno-sis as determined by transesophageal echocardiography. Am J Cardiol. 2009;103(5):713–7. doi:10.1016/j.amjcard.2008.11.026. S0002-9149(08)02023-7 [pii].

85. Avegliano G, Evangelista A, Elorz C, Gonzalez-Alujas T, Garcia del Castillo H, Soler-Soler J. Acute peripheral arterial ischemia and suspected aortic dissection: usefulness of transesophageal

echocardiography in differential diagnosis with aortic thrombosis. Am J Cardiol. 2002;90(6):674–7. doi:S0002914902025857 [pii].

86. Gottsegen JM, Coplan NL. The atherosclerotic aortic arch: considerations in diagnostic imaging. Prev Cardiol. 2008;11(3): 162–7.

87. Wareing TH, Davila-Roman VG, Barzilai B, Murphy SF, Kouchoukos NT. Management of the severely atherosclerotic ascending aorta during cardiac operations. A strategy for detection and treatment. J Thorac Cardiovasc Surg. 1992;103(3):453–62.

88. Corti R. Noninvasive imaging of atherosclerotic vessels by MRI for clinical assessment of the effectiveness of therapy. Pharmacol Ther. 2006;110(1):57–70. doi:10.1016/j.pharmthera.2005.09.004.

89. Kronzon I. Protruding aortic atheroma: is there a need for a new imaging modality? Isr Med Assoc J. 2000;2(1):54–5.

90. Tahara N, Kai H, Ishibashi M, Nakaura H, Kaida H, Baba K, Hayabuchi N, Imaizumi T. Simvastatin attenuates plaque inflammation: evaluation by fluorodeoxyglucose positron emission tomography. J Am Coll Cardiol. 2006;48(9):1825–31. doi:10.1016/j.jacc.2006.03.069. S0735-1097(06)01979-6 [pii].

91. Kumral E, Balkir K, Yagdi T, Kara E, Evyapan D, Bilkay O. Microembolic signals in patients undergoing coronary artery bypass grafting. Effect of aortic atherosclerosis. Tex Heart Inst J. 2001;28(1):16–20.

92. Viguier A, Pavy le Traon A, Massabuau P, Valton L, Larrue V. Asymptomatic cerebral embolic signals in patients with acute cerebral ischaemia and severe aortic arch atherosclerosis. J Neurol. 2001;248(9):768–71.

93. Khatri IA, Mian N, Alkawi A, Janjua N, Kirmani JF, Saric M, Levine JC, Qureshi AI. Catheter-based aortography fails to identify aortic atherosclerotic lesions detected on transesophageal echocardiography. J Neuroimaging. 2005;15(3):261–5. doi:10.1177/1051228405277344.

94. Goldstein LB, Adams R, Alberts MJ, Appel LJ, Brass LM, Bushnell CD, Culebras A, DeGraba TJ, Gorelick PB, Guyton JR, Hart RG, Howard G, Kelly-Hayes M, Nixon JV, Sacco RL. Primary prevention of ischemic stroke: a guideline from the American Heart Association/American Stroke Association Stroke Council: cosponsored by the Atherosclerotic Peripheral Vascular Disease Interdisciplinary Working Group; Cardiovascular Nursing Council; Clinical Cardiology Council; Nutrition, Physical Activity, and Metabolism Council; and the

Quality of Care and Outcomes Research Interdisciplinary Working Group. Circulation. 2006;113(24):e873–923. doi:10.1161/01.STR.0000223048.70103.F1. 113/24/e873 [pii].

95. Yonemura A, Momiyama Y, Fayad ZA, Ayaori M, Ohmori R, Kihara T, Tanaka N, Nakaya K, Ogura M, Taniguchi H, Kusuhara M, Nagata M, Nakamura H, Tamai S, Ohsuzu F. Effect of lipid-lowering therapy with atorvastatin on atherosclerotic aortic plaques: a 2-year follow-up by noninvasive MRI. Eur J Cardiovasc Prev Rehabil. 2009;16(2):222–8. doi:10.1097/HJR.0b013e32832948a0.

96. Corti R, Fayad ZA, Fuster V, Worthley SG, Helft G, Chesebro J, Mercuri M, Badimon JJ. Effects of lipid-lowering by simvastatin on human atherosclerotic lesions: a longitudinal study by high-resolution, noninvasive magnetic resonance imaging. Circulation. 2001;104(3):249–52.

97. Corti R, Fuster V, Fayad ZA, Worthley SG, Helft G, Smith D, Weinberger J, Wentzel J, Mizsei G, Mercuri M, Badimon JJ. Lipid lowering by simvastatin induces regression of human atherosclerotic lesions: two years' follow-up by high-resolution noninvasive magnetic resonance imaging. Circulation. 2002;106(23):2884–7.

98. Corti R, Fuster V, Fayad ZA, Worthley SG, Helft G, Chaplin WF, Muntwyler J, Viles-Gonzalez JF, Weinberger J, Smith DA, Mizsei G, Badimon JJ. Effects of aggressive versus conventional lipid-lowering therapy by simvastatin on human atherosclerotic lesions: a prospective, randomized, double-blind trial with high-resolution magnetic resonance imaging. J Am Coll Cardiol. 2005;46(1):106–12. doi:10.1016/j.jacc.2005.03.054.

99. Yonemura A, Momiyama Y, Fayad ZA, Ayaori M, Ohmori R, Higashi K, Kihara T, Sawada S, Iwamoto N, Ogura M, Taniguchi H, Kusuhara M, Nagata M, Nakamura H, Tamai S, Ohsuzu F. Effect of lipid-lowering therapy with atorvastatin on athero-sclerotic aortic plaques detected by noninvasive magnetic reso-nance imaging. J Am Coll Cardiol. 2005;45(5):733–42. doi:10.1016/j.jacc.2004.11.039. S0735-1097(04)02397-6 [pii].

100. Smith Jr SC, Allen J, Blair SN, Bonow RO, Brass LM, Fonarow GC, Grundy SM, Hiratzka L, Jones D, Krumholz HM, Mosca L, Pearson T, Pfeffer MA, Taubert KA. AHA/ACC guidelines for secondary prevention for patients with coronary and other atherosclerotic vascular disease: 2006 update endorsed by the National Heart, Lung, and Blood Institute. J Am Coll Cardiol. 2006;47(10):2130–9. doi:10.1016/j.jacc.2006.04.026. S0735-1097(06)01043-6 [pii].

101. Hiratzka LF, Bakris GL, Beckman JA, Bersin RM, Carr VF, Casey Jr DE, Eagle KA, Hermann LK, Isselbacher EM, Kazerooni EA, Kouchoukos NT, Lytle BW, Milewicz DM, Reich DL, Sen S, Shinn JA, Svensson LG, Williams DM. 2010 ACCF/AHA/AATS/ACR/ASA/SCA/SCAI/SIR/STS/SVM guidelines for the diagnosis and management of patients with Thoracic Aortic Disease: a report of the American College of Cardiology Foundation/American Heart Association Task Force on Practice Guidelines, American Association for Thoracic Surgery, American College of Radiology, American Stroke Association, Society of Cardiovascular Anesthesiologists, Society for Cardiovascular Angiography and Interventions, Society of Interventional Radiology, Society of Thoracic Surgeons, and Society for Vascular Medicine. Circulation. 2010;121(13):e266–369. doi:10.1161/CIR.0b013e3181d4739e. CIR.0b013e3181d4739e [pii].

102. Kernan WN, Ovbiagele B, Black HR, Bravata DM, Chimowitz MI, Ezekowitz MD, Fang MC, Fisher M, Furie KL, Heck DV, Johnston SC, Kasner SE, Kittner SJ, Mitchell PH, Rich MW, Richardson D, Schwamm LH, Wilson JA. Guidelines for the Prevention of Stroke in Patients with Stroke and Transient Ischemic Attack: a guideline for Healthcare Professionals from the American Heart Association/American Stroke Association. Stroke. 2014. doi:10.1161/STR.0000000000000024.

103. Stone NJ, Robinson J, Lichtenstein AH, Merz CN, Blum CB, Eckel RH, Goldberg AC, Gordon D, Levy D, Lloyd-Jones DM, McBride P, Schwartz JS, Shero ST, Smith Jr SC, Watson K, Wilson PW. 2013 ACC/AHA Guideline on the Treatment of Blood Cholesterol to Reduce Atherosclerotic Cardiovascular Risk in Adults: a report of the American College of Cardiology/American Heart Association Task Force on Practice Guidelines. Circulation. 2013. doi:10.1161/01.cir.0000437738.63853.7a. 01.cir.0000437738.63853.7a [pii].

104. Nakagawa K, Hirai T, Sakurai K, Ohara K, Nozawa T, Inoue H. Thoracic aortic plaque enhances hypercoagulability in patients with nonrheumatic atrial fibrillation. Circ J. 2007;71(1):52–6.

105. Nakagawa K, Hirai T, Shinokawa N, Takashima S, Nozawa T, Asanoi H, Inoue H. Aortic spontaneous echocardiographic contrast and hemostatic markers in patients with nonrheumatic atrial fibrillation. Chest. 2002;121(2):500–5.

106. Ferrari E, Vidal R, Chevallier T, Baudouy M. Atherosclerosis of the thoracic aorta and aortic debris as a marker of poor

prognosis: benefit of oral anticoagulants. J Am Coll Cardiol. 1999;33(5):1317–22.

107. Bruns FJ, Segel DP, Adler S. Control of cholesterol emboliza-tion by discontinuation of anticoagulant therapy. Am J Med Sci. 1978;275(1):105–8.

108. Blackshear JL, Jahangir A, Oldenburg WA, Safford RE. Digital embolization from plaque-related thrombus in the thoracic aorta: identification with transesophageal echocardiography and resolution with warfarin therapy. Mayo Clin Proc. 1993; 68(3):268–72.

109. Dahlberg PJ, Frecentese DF, Cogbill TH. Cholesterol embolism: experience with 22 histologically proven cases. Surgery. 1989;105(6):737–46. doi:0039-6060(89)90333-4 [pii].

110. Hausmann D, Gulba D, Bargheer K, Niedermeyer J, Comess KA, Daniel WG. Successful thrombolysis of an aortic-arch thrombus in a patient after mesenteric embolism. N Engl J Med. 1992;327(7):500–1. doi:10.1056/NEJM199208133270717.

111. Blackshear JL, Zabalgoitia M, Pennock G, Fenster P, Strauss R, Halperin J, Asinger R, Pearce LA. Warfarin safety and efficacy in patients with thoracic aortic plaque and atrial fibrillation. SPAF TEE Investigators. Stroke Prevention and Atrial Fibrillation. Transesophageal echocardiography. Am J Cardiol. 1999;83(3):453–455, A459. doi:S0002914998008868 [pii].

112. Trial C. Aortic Arch Related Cerebral Hazard Trial (ARCH). 2005.

113. Tsilimparis N, Hanack U, Pisimisis G, Yousefi S, Wintzer C, Ruckert RI. Thrombus in the non-aneurysmal, non-atherosclerotic descending thoracic aorta – an unusual source of arterial embolism. Eur J Vasc Endovasc Surg. 2011;41(4):450–7. doi:10.1016/j.ejvs.2010.11.004. S1078-5884(10)00681-7 [pii].

114. Pagni S, Trivedi J, Ganzel BL, Williams M, Kapoor N, Ross C, Slater AD. Thoracic aortic mobile thrombus: is there a role for early surgical intervention? Ann Thorac Surg. 2011;91(6):1875–81. doi:10.1016/j.athoracsur.2011.02.011. S0003-4975(11)00435-8 [pii].

115. Martens T, Van Herzeele I, Jacobs B, De Ryck F, Randon C, Vermassen F. Treatment of symptomatic mobile aortic throm-bus. Acta Chir Belg. 2010;110(3):361–4.

116. Soleimani A, Marzban M, Sahebjam M, Shirani S, Sotoudeh-Anvari M, Abbasi A. Floating thrombus in the aortic arch as an origin of simultaneous peripheral emboli. J Card Surg. 2008;23(6):762–4. doi:10.1111/j.1540-8191.2008.00694.x. JCS694 [pii].

117. Berneder S, van Ingen G, Eigel P. Arch thrombus formation in an apparently normal aorta as a source for recurrent peripheral embolization. Thorac Cardiovasc Surg. 2006;54(8):548–9. doi:10.1055/s-2006-923976.

118. Taglietti L, Pontoglio S, Di Flumeri G, EP R, Vettoretto N, Ghilardi G, Barozzi G, Poiatti R, Giovanetti M. Acute thrombosis of abdominal aorta and hypercoagulable disorders. Int Angiol. 2008;27(2):157–65.

119. Marcu CB, Donohue TJ, Ghantous AE. Spontaneous aortic thrombosis and embolization: antithrombin deficiency and the work-up of hypercoagulable states. CMAJ. 2005;173(9):1027–9. doi:10.1503/cmaj.050464. 173/9/1027 [pii].

120. Kotani S, Hattori K, Kato Y, Shibata T. Thrombus in the distal aortic arch after apicoaortic conduit for severe aortic stenosis. Interact Cardiovasc Thorac Surg. 2010;10(3):486–8. doi:10.1510/icvts.2009.220707. icvts.2009.220707 [pii].

121. Chin SO, Lee JJ, Hwang YH, Han JJ, Maeng CH, Baek SK, Choi CW. Aortic thrombosis resolved with enoxaparin in a patient treated with cisplatin-based regimen for small cell lung cancer. Int J Hematol. 2010;91(5):892–6. doi:10.1007/s12185-010-0571-3.

122. Stordiau GE, Alecha JS, Goni S, Zozaya JM, Centeno R, Tricas JM. Arterial thromboembolism from aortic floating thrombus in a patient with Crohn's disease. J Crohns Colitis. 2011;5(2):169–70. doi:10.1016/j.crohns.2011.01.002. S1873-9946(11)00033-X [pii].

123. Sanon S, Phung MK, Lentz R, Buja LM, Tung PP, McPherson DD, Fuentes F. Floating, non-occlusive, mobile aortic thrombus and splenic infarction associated with protein C deficiency. J Am Soc Echocardiogr. 2009;22(12):1419.e1411–3. doi:10.1016/j.echo.2009.06.004. S0894-7317(09)00575-6 [pii].

124. Sohn V, Arthurs Z, Andersen C, Starnes B. Aortic thrombus due to essential thrombocytosis: strategies for medical and surgical management. Ann Vasc Surg. 2008;22(5):676–80. doi:10.1016/j.avsg.2007.12.018. S0890-5096(08)00079-4 [pii].

125. Loffroy R, Boussel L, Farhat F, Douek P. Isolated floating thrombus of the thoracic aorta: a rare sign of traumatic aortic injury managed with anticoagulant therapy. Ann Thorac Surg. 2007;84(5):1766. doi:10.1016/j.athoracsur.2006.10.078. S0003-4975(06)02117-5 [pii].

126. Chatterjee S, Eagle SS, Adler DH, Byrne JG. Incidental discovery of an ascending aortic thrombus: should this patient undergo

surgical intervention? J Thorac Cardiovasc Surg. 2010;140(1):e14–6. doi:10.1016/j.jtcvs.2009.07.010. S0022-5223(09)00915-5 [pii].

127. Fanelli F, Gazzetti M, Boatta E, Ruggiero M, Lucatelli P, Speziale F. Acute left arm ischemia associated with floating thrombus in the proximal descending aorta: combined endovascular and surgical therapy. Cardiovasc Intervent Radiol. 2011;34(1):193–7. doi:10.1007/s00270-010-9804-3.

128. Hisagi M, Morota T, Endo M, Taketani T, Takamoto S. Floating thrombus in the ascending aorta. Gen Thorac Cardiovasc Surg. 2007;55(1):38–40.

129. Boufi M, Mameli A, Compes P, Hartung O, Alimi YS. Elective stent-graft treatment for the management of thoracic aorta mural thrombus. Eur J Vasc Endovasc Surg. 2014;47(4):335–41. doi:10.1016/j.ejvs.2013.11.014. S1078-5884(13)00733-8 [pii].

130. Luebke T, Aleksic M, Brunkwall J. Endovascular therapy of a symptomatic mobile thrombus of the thoracic aorta. Eur J Vasc Endovasc Surg. 2008;36(5):550–2. doi:10.1016/j.ejvs.2008.07.004. S1078-5884(08)00398-5 [pii].

131. Scott DJ, White JM, Arthurs ZM. Endovascular management of a mobile thoracic aortic thrombus following recurrent distal thromboembolism: a case report and literature review. Vasc Endovascular Surg. 2014;48(3):246–50. doi:10.1177/1538574413513845. 1538574413513845 [pii].

132. Mahnken AH, Hoffman A, Autschbach R, Damberg AL. Bare metal stenting for endovascular exclusion of aortic arch thrombi. Cardiovasc Intervent Radiol. 2013;36(4):1127–31. doi:10.1007/s00270-013-0566-6.

133. Metsemakers WJ, Duchateau J, Vanhoenacker F, Tielemans Y, De Leersnyder J. Floating aortic thrombus: the endovascular approach. Acta Chir Belg. 2013;113(1):47–50.

134. Wolf PS, Burman HE, Starnes BW. Endovascular treatment of massive thoracic aortic thrombus and associated ruptured atheroma. Ann Vasc Surg. 2010;24(3):416.e9–416.e12. doi:10.1016/j.avsg.2009.10.004.

135. Alhan C, Karabulut H, Senay S, Cagil H, Toraman F. Endovascular treatment of occlusive abdominal aortic thrombosis. Heart Vessels. 2010;25(1):70–2. doi:10.1007/s00380-009-1169-7.

136. Piffaretti G, Tozzi M, Caronno R, Castelli P. Endovascular treatment for mobile thrombus of the thoracic aorta. Eur J Cardiothorac Surg. 2007;32(4):664–6. doi:10.1016/j.ejcts.2007.06.043. S1010-7940(07)00607-0 [pii].

137. Fueglistaler P, Wolff T, Guerke L, Stierli P, Eugster T. Endovascular stent graft for symptomatic mobile thrombus of the thoracic aorta. J Vasc Surg. 2005;42(4):781–3. doi:10.1016/j. jvs.2005.05.054. S0741-5214(05)00974-2 [pii].

138. Nakajima M, Tsuchiya K, Honda Y, Koshiyama H, Kobayashi T. Acute pulmonary embolism after cerebral infarction associated with a mobile thrombus in the ascending aorta. Gen Thorac Cardiovasc Surg. 2009;57(12):654–6. doi:10.1007/ s11748-009-0444-y.

139. Bockler D, von Tengg-Kobligk H, Schoebinger M, Gross ML, Schumacher H, Ockert S, Allenberg JR. An unusual cause of peripheral artery embolism: floating thrombus of the thoracic aorta surgically removed. Vasa. 2007;36(2):121–3.

140. Krishnamoorthy V, Bhatt K, Nicolau R, Borhani M, Schwartz DE. Transesophageal echocardiography-guided aortic thrombectomy in a patient with a mobile thoracic aortic thrombus. Semin Cardiothorac Vasc Anesth. 2011;15(4):176–8. doi:10.1177/1089253211415123. 1089253211415123 [pii].

141. Josephson GD, Tiefenbrun J, Harvey J. Thrombosis of the descending thoracic aorta: a case report. Surgery. 1993;114(3):598–600. doi:0039-6060(93)90300-3 [pii].

142. Kalangos A, Baldovinos A, Vuille C, Montessuit M, Faidutti B. Floating thrombus in the ascending aorta: a rare cause of peripheral emboli. J Vasc Surg. 1997;26(1):150–4. doi:S0741-5214(97)70161-7 [pii].

143. Sawada T, Shimokawa T. Giant thrombus in the ascending aorta that caused systemic embolism. Interact Cardiovasc Thorac Surg. 2011;12(6):1048–50. doi:10.1510/icvts.2011.266445. icvts.2011.266445 [pii].

144. Calderon P, Heredero A, Pastor A, Higueras J, Hernandez J, Karagounis PA, Aldamiz-Echevarria G. Successful removal of a floating thrombus in ascending aorta. Ann Thorac Surg. 2011;91(5):e67–9. doi:10.1016/j.athoracsur.2010.12.011. S0003-4975(10)02788-8 [pii].

145. Namura O, Sogawa M, Asami F, Okamoto T, Hanzawa K, Hayashi J. Floating thrombus originating from an almost normal thoracic aorta. Gen Thorac Cardiovasc Surg. 2011;59(9):612–5. doi:10.1007/s11748-010-0752-2.

146. Tunick PA, Culliford AT, Lamparello PJ, Kronzon I. Atheromatosis of the aortic arch as an occult source of multiple systemic emboli. Ann Intern Med. 1991;114(5):391–2.

147. Iyer AP, Sadasivan D, Kamal U, Sharma S. Resolution of large intra-aortic thrombus following anticoagulation therapy. Heart Lung Circ. 2009;18(1):49–50. doi:10.1016/j.hlc.2007.09.006. S1443-9506(07)00900-6 [pii].

148. Pousios D, Velissaris T, Duggan S, Tsang G. Floating intra-aortic thrombus presenting as distal arterial embolism. Interact Cardiovasc Thorac Surg. 2009;9(3):532–4. doi:10.1510/ icvts.2009.206268. icvts.2009.206268 [pii].

149. Fayad ZY, Semaan E, Fahoum B, Briggs M, Tortolani A, D'Ayala M. Aortic mural thrombus in the normal or minimally atherosclerotic aorta. Ann Vasc Surg. 2013;27(3):282–90. doi:10.1016/j.avsg.2012.03.011. S0890-5096(12)00258-0 [pii].

150. Kruger T, Liske B, Ziemer S, Lindemann S, Ziemer G. Thrombolysis to treat thrombi of the aortic arch. Clin Appl Thromb Hemost. 2011;17(4):340–5. doi:10.1177/1076029610364519. 1076029610364519 [pii].

151. Durdil V, Fiedler J, Alan D, Vejvoda J, Veselka J. Multiple mobile aortic thrombosis treated by thrombolysis. A case report. J Thromb Thrombolysis. 2007;24(3):315–6. doi:10.1007/ s11239-007-0091-z.

152. Bays HE, Dujovne CA. Drug interactions of lipid-altering drugs. Drug Saf. 1998;19(5):355–71.

153. Farmer JA, Gotto Jr AM. Antihyperlipidaemic agents. Drug interactions of clinical significance. Drug Saf. 1994;11(5):301–9.

154. Pan HY, DeVault AR, Swites BJ, Whigan D, Ivashkiv E, Willard DA, Brescia D. Pharmacokinetics and pharmacodynamics of pravastatin alone and with cholestyramine in hypercholesterolemia. Clin Pharmacol Ther. 1990;48(2):201–7. doi:0009-9236(90)90152-U [pii].

155. Nakai A, Nishikata M, Matsuyama K, Ichikawa M. Drug interaction between simvastatin and cholestyramine in vitro and in vivo. Biol Pharm Bull. 1996;19(9):1231–3.

156. Smith HT, Jokubaitis LA, Troendle AJ, Hwang DS, Robinson WT. Pharmacokinetics of fluvastatin and specific drug interactions. Am J Hypertens. 1993;6(11 Pt 2):375S–82. doi:0895-7061(93)90482-2 [pii].

157. Richter WO, Jacob BG, Schwandt P. Interaction between fibre and lovastatin. Lancet. 1991;338(8768):706.

158. Martin PD, Schneck DW, Dane AL, Warwick MJ. The effect of a combination antacid preparation containing aluminium hydroxide and magnesium hydroxide on rosuvastatin pharmacokinetics. Curr Med Res Opin. 2008;24(4):1231–5. doi:10.1185/ 030079908X280662. 4355 [pii].

159. Langtry HD, Markham A. Fluvastatin: a review of its use in lipid disorders. Drugs. 1999;57(4):583–606.

160. Plosker GL, Wagstaff AJ. Fluvastatin: a review of its pharmacology and use in the management of hypercholesterolaemia. Drugs. 1996;51(3):433–59.

161. Pan HY, DeVault AR, Brescia D, Willard DA, McGovern ME, Whigan DB, Ivashkiv E. Effect of food on pravastatin pharmacokinetics and pharmacodynamics. Int J Clin Pharmacol Ther Toxicol. 1993;31(6):291–4.

162. Deslypere JP. Clinical implications of the biopharmaceutical properties of fluvastatin. Am J Cardiol. 1994;73(14):12D–7.

163. Radulovic LL, Cilla DD, Posvar EL, Sedman AJ, Whitfield LR. Effect of food on the bioavailability of atorvastatin, an HMG-CoA reductase inhibitor. J Clin Pharmacol. 1995;35(10):990–4.

164. Lennernas H, Fager G. Pharmacodynamics and pharmacokinetics of the HMG-CoA reductase inhibitors. Similarities and differences. Clin Pharmacokinet. 1997;32(5):403–25. doi:10.2165/00003088-199732050-00005.

165. Izzo AA, Di Carlo G, Borrelli F, Ernst E. Cardiovascular pharmacotherapy and herbal medicines: the risk of drug interaction. Int J Cardiol. 2005;98(1):1–14. doi:10.1016/j.ijcard.2003.06.039. S0167527303006272 [pii].

166. Williams D, Feely J. Pharmacokinetic-pharmacodynamic drug interactions with HMG-CoA reductase inhibitors. Clin Pharmacokinet. 2002;41(5):343–70. doi:10.2165/00003088-200241050-00003.

167. Kim J, Ahn BJ, Chae HS, Han S, Doh K, Choi J, Jun YK, Lee YW, Yim DS. A population pharmacokinetic-pharmacodynamic model for simvastatin that predicts low-density lipoprotein-cholesterol reduction in patients with primary hyperlipidaemia. Basic Clin Pharmacol Toxicol. 2011;109(3):156–63. doi:10.1111/j.1742-7843.2011.00700.x.

168. Wenaweser P, Eshtehardi P, Abrecht L, Zwahlen M, Schmidlin K, Windecker S, Meier B, Haeberli A, Hess OM. A randomised determination of the Effect of Fluvastatin and Atorvastatin on top of dual antiplatelet treatment on platelet aggregation after implantation of coronary drug-eluting stents. The EFA-Trial. Thromb Haemost. 2010;104(3):554–62. doi:10.1160/TH09-11-0765. 09-11-0765 [pii].

169. Geisler T, Zurn C, Paterok M, Gohring-Frischholz K, Bigalke B, Stellos K, Seizer P, Kraemer BF, Dippon J, May AE, Herdeg C, Gawaz M. Statins do not adversely affect post-interventional residual platelet aggregation and outcomes in patients under-

going coronary stenting treated by dual antiplatelet therapy. Eur Heart J. 2008;29(13):1635–43. doi:10.1093/eurheartj/ehn212. ehn212 [pii].

170. Dinicolantonio JJ, Serebruany VL. Exploring the ticagrelor-statin interplay in the PLATO trial. Cardiology. 2013;124(2):105–7. doi:10.1159/000346151.

171. Teng R, Mitchell PD, Butler KA. Pharmacokinetic interaction studies of co-administration of ticagrelor and atorvastatin or simvastatin in healthy volunteers. Eur J Clin Pharmacol. 2013;69(3):477–87. doi:10.1007/s00228-012-1369-4.

172. Neuvonen PJ, Kantola T, Kivisto KT. Simvastatin but not pravastatin is very susceptible to interaction with the CYP3A4 inhibitor itraconazole. Clin Pharmacol Ther. 1998;63(3):332–41. doi:10.1016/S0009-9236(98)90165-5.

173. Horn M. Coadministration of itraconazole with hypolipidemic agents may induce rhabdomyolysis in healthy individuals. Arch Dermatol. 1996;132(10):1254.

174. Goldberg R, Roth D. Evaluation of fluvastatin in the treatment of hypercholesterolemia in renal transplant recipients taking cyclosporine. Transplantation. 1996;62(11):1559–64.

175. McKenney JM. Efficacy and safety of rosuvastatin in treatment of dyslipidemia. Am J Health Syst Pharm. 2005;62(10):1033–47.

176. Athyros VG, Mikhailidis DP, Papageorgiou AA, Bouloukos VI, Pehlivanidis AN, Symeonidis AN, Kakafika AI, Daskalopoulou SS, Elisaf M. Effect of statins and aspirin alone and in combination on clinical outcome in dyslipidaemic patients with coronary heart disease. A subgroup analysis of the GREACE study. Platelets. 2005;16(2):65–71. doi:10.1080/09537100400009321. VG477N1368450605 [pii].

177. Angiolillo DJ, Alfonso F. Clopidogrel-statin interaction: myth or reality? J Am Coll Cardiol. 2007;50(4):296–8. doi:10.1016/j.jacc.2007.04.041. S0735-1097(07)01471-4 [pii].

178. Steinhubl SR, Akers WS. Clopidogrel-statin interaction: a mountain or a mole hill? Am Heart J. 2006;152(2):200–3. doi:10.1016/j.ahj.2006.01.001. S0002-8703(06)00051-2 [pii].

179. Tafreshi MJ, Zagnoni LG, Gentry EJ. Combination of clopidogrel and statins: a hypothetical interaction or therapeutic dilemma? Pharmacotherapy. 2006;26(3):388–94. doi:10.1592/phco.26.3.388.

180. Blagojevic A, Delancy JA, Levesque LE, Dendukuri N, Boivin JF, Brophy JM. Investigation of an interaction between statins and clopidogrel after percutaneous coronary intervention: a

cohort study. Pharmacoepidemiol Drug Saf. 2009;18(5):362–9. doi:10.1002/pds.1716.

181. Shen J, Zhang RY, Zhang Q. Impact of statins on clopidogrel platelet inhibition in patients with acute coronary syndrome or stable angina. Zhonghua Xin Xue Guan Bing Za Zhi. 2008;36(9):807–11.

182. Bhindi R, Ormerod O, Newton J, Banning AP, Testa L. Interaction between statins and clopidogrel: is there anything clinically relevant? QJM. 2008;101(12):915–25. doi:10.1093/qjmed/hcn089. hcn089 [pii].

183. Zurn CS, Geisler T, Paterok M, Gawaz M. Influence of statins on the antiplatelet effect of clopidogrel and on cardiovascular outcome in patients after coronary intervention. Dtsch Med Wochenschr. 2008;133(16):817–22. doi:10.1055/s-2008-1075654.

184. Trenk D, Hochholzer W, Frundi D, Stratz C, Valina CM, Bestehorn HP, Buttner HJ, Neumann FJ. Impact of cytochrome P450 3A4-metabolized statins on the antiplatelet effect of a 600-mg loading dose clopidogrel and on clinical outcome in patients undergoing elective coronary stent placement. Thromb Haemost. 2008;99(1):174–81. doi:10.1160/TH07-08-0503. 08010174 [pii].

185. Han YL, Li CY, Li Y, Kang J, Yan CH. The antiplatelet effect of clopidogrel is not attenuated by statin treatment in patients with acute coronary syndromes undergone coronary stenting. Zhonghua Xin Xue Guan Bing Za Zhi. 2007;35(9):788–92.

186. Saw J, Brennan DM, Steinhubl SR, Bhatt DL, Mak KH, Fox K, Topol EJ. Lack of evidence of a clopidogrel-statin interaction in the CHARISMA trial. J Am Coll Cardiol. 2007;50(4):291–5. doi:10.1016/j.jacc.2007.01.097. S0735-1097(07)01474-X [pii].

187. Serebruany VL, Midei MG, Malinin AI, Oshrine BR, Lowry DR, Sane DC, Tanguay JF, Steinhubl SR, Berger PB, O'Connor CM, Hennekens CH. Absence of interaction between atorvastatin or other statins and clopidogrel: results from the interaction study. Arch Intern Med. 2004;164(18):2051–7. doi:10.1001/archinte.164.18.2051. 164/18/2051 [pii].

188. Wienbergen H, Gitt AK, Schiele R, Juenger C, Heer T, Meisenzahl C, Limbourg P, Bossaller C, Senges J. Comparison of clinical benefits of clopidogrel therapy in patients with acute coronary syndromes taking atorvastatin versus other statin therapies. Am J Cardiol. 2003;92(3):285–8. doi:S000291490300626X [pii].

189. Serebruany VL, Malinin AI, Callahan KP, Gurbel PA, Steinhubl SR. Statins do not affect platelet inhibition with clopidogrel

during coronary stenting. Atherosclerosis. 2001;159(1):239–41. doi:S0021915001006062 [pii].

190. Wenaweser P, Windecker S, Billinger M, Cook S, Togni M, Meier B, Haeberli A, Hess OM. Effect of atorvastatin and pravastatin on platelet inhibition by aspirin and clopidogrel treatment in patients with coronary stent thrombosis. Am J Cardiol. 2007;99(3):353–6. doi:10.1016/j.amjcard.2006.08.036. S0002-9149(06)02061-3 [pii].

191. Gulec S, Ozdol C, Rahimov U, Atmaca Y, Kumbasar D, Erol C. Myonecrosis after elective percutaneous coronary intervention: effect of clopidogrel-statin interaction. J Invasive Cardiol. 2005;17(11):589–93.

192. Neubauer H, Gunesdogan B, Hanefeld C, Spiecker M, Mugge A. Lipophilic statins interfere with the inhibitory effects of clopidogrel on platelet function – a flow cytometry study. Eur Heart J. 2003;24(19):1744–9. doi:S0195668X03004421 [pii].

193. Mukherjee D, Kline-Rogers E, Fang J, Munir K, Eagle KA. Lack of clopidogrel-CYP3A4 statin interaction in patients with acute coronary syndrome. Heart. 2005;91(1):23–6. doi:10.1136/hrt.2004.035014. 91/1/23 [pii].

194. Mach F, Senouf D, Fontana P, Boehlen F, Reber G, Daali Y, de Moerloose P, Sigwart U. Not all statins interfere with clopidogrel during antiplatelet therapy. Eur J Clin Invest. 2005;35(8):476–81. doi:10.1111/j.1365-2362.2005.01522.x. ECI1522 [pii].

195. Smith SM, Judge HM, Peters G, Storey RF. Multiple antiplatelet effects of clopidogrel are not modulated by statin type in patients undergoing percutaneous coronary intervention. Platelets. 2004;15(8):465–74. doi:10.1080/0953710412331272532. YR2F8RXTTGNJNND1 [pii].

196. Ojeifo O, Wiviott SD, Antman EM, Murphy SA, Udell JA, Bates ER, Mega JL, Sabatine MS, O'Donoghue ML. Concomitant administration of clopidogrel with statins or calcium channel blockers: insights from the TRITON-TIMI 38 (trial to assess improvement in therapeutic outcomes by optimizing platelet inhibition with prasugrel-thrombolysis in myocardial infarction 38) trial. J Am Coll Cardiol Intv. 2013. doi:10.1016/j.jcin.2013.06.014.

197. Farid NA, Small DS, Payne CD, Jakubowski JA, Brandt JT, Li YG, Ernest CS, Salazar DE, Konkoy CS, Winters KJ. Effect of atorvastatin on the pharmacokinetics and pharmacodynamics of prasugrel and clopidogrel in healthy subjects.

Pharmacotherapy.   2008;28(12):1483–94.   doi:10.1592/phco.28.12.1483.

198. Holbrook AM, Pereira JA, Labiris R, McDonald H, Douketis JD, Crowther M, Wells PS. Systematic overview of warfarin and its drug and food interactions. Arch Intern Med. 2005;165(10):1095–106. doi:10.1001/archinte.165.10.1095.

199. Nutescu E, Chuatrisorn I, Hellenbart E. Drug and dietary interactions of warfarin and novel oral anticoagulants: an update. J Thromb Thrombolysis. 2011;31(3):326–43. doi:10.1007/s11239-011-0561-1.

200. Black DJ, Kunze KL, Wienkers LC, Gidal BE, Seaton TL, McDonnell ND, Evans JS, Bauwens JE, Trager WF. Warfarin-fluconazole. II. A metabolically based drug interaction: in vivo studies. Drug Metab Dispos. 1996;24(4):422–8.

201. Hemeryck A, De Vriendt C, Belpaire FM. Inhibition of CYP2C9 by selective serotonin reuptake inhibitors: in vitro studies with tolbutamide and (S)-warfarin using human liver microsomes. Eur J Clin Pharmacol. 1999;54(12):947–51.

202. Izzo AA, Ernst E. Interactions between herbal medicines and prescribed drugs: an updated systematic review. Drugs. 2009;69(13):1777–98. doi:10.2165/11317010-000000000-00000.

203. Westergren T, Johansson P, Molden E. Probable warfarin-simvastatin interaction. Ann Pharmacother. 2007;41(7):1292–5. doi:10.1345/aph.1K167.

204. Tadros R, Shakib S. Warfarin – indications, risks and drug interactions. Aust Fam Physician. 2010;39(7):476–9.

205. Ghaswalla PK, Harpe SE, Tassone D, Slattum PW. Warfarin-antibiotic interactions in older adults of an outpatient anticoagulation clinic. Am J Geriatr Pharmacother. 2012;10(6):352–60. doi:10.1016/j.amjopharm.2012.09.006.

206. Rice PJ, Perry RJ, Afzal Z, Stockley IH. Antibacterial prescribing and warfarin: a review. Br Dent J. 2003;194(8):411–5. doi:10.1038/sj.bdj.4810049.

207. Abernethy DR, Kaminsky LS, Dickinson TH. Selective inhibition of warfarin metabolism by diltiazem in humans. J Pharmacol Exp Ther. 1991;257(1):411–5.

208. Yamazaki H, Shimada T. Comparative studies of in vitro inhibition of cytochrome P450 3A4-dependent testosterone 6beta-hydroxylation by roxithromycin and its metabolites, troleandomycin, and erythromycin. Drug Metab Dispos. 1998;26(11):1053–7.

209. Randinitis EJ, Alvey CW, Koup JR, Rausch G, Abel R, Bron NJ, Hounslow NJ, Vassos AB, Sedman AJ. Drug interactions with

clinafloxacin. Antimicrob Agents Chemother. 2001;45(9): 2543–52.

210. Heimark LD, Wienkers L, Kunze K, Gibaldi M, Eddy AC, Trager WF, O'Reilly RA, Goulart DA. The mechanism of the interaction between amiodarone and warfarin in humans. Clin Pharmacol Ther. 1992;51(4):398–407.

211. O'Reilly RA, Trager WF, Rettie AE, Goulart DA. Interaction of amiodarone with racemic warfarin and its separated enantiomorphs in humans. Clin Pharmacol Ther. 1987;42(3):290–4. doi:0009-9236(87)90150-0 [pii].

212. Rettie AE, Jones JP. Clinical and toxicological relevance of CYP2C9: drug-drug interactions and pharmacogenetics. Annu Rev Pharmacol Toxicol. 2005;45:477–94. doi:10.1146/annurev. pharmtox.45.120403.095821.

213. Van Booven D, Marsh S, McLeod H, Carrillo MW, Sangkuhl K, Klein TE, Altman RB. Cytochrome P450 2C9-CYP2C9. Pharmacogenet Genomics. 2010;20(4):277–81. doi:10.1097/ FPC.0b013e3283349e84.

214. Samer CF, Lorenzini KI, Rollason V, Daali Y, Desmeules JA. Applications of CYP450 testing in the clinical setting. Mol Diagn Ther. 2013;17(3):165–84. doi:10.1007/s40291-013-0028-5.

215. Nathisuwan S, Dilokthornsakul P, Chaiyakunapruk N, Morarai T, Yodting T, Piriyachananusorn N. Assessing evidence of interaction between smoking and warfarin: a systematic review and meta-analysis. Chest. 2011;139(5):1130–9. doi:10.1378/chest.10-0777. 139/5/1130 [pii].

216. Hersh EV, Moore PA. Drug interactions in dentistry: the importance of knowing your CYPs. J Am Dent Assoc. 2004;135(3):298–311.

217. Hijazi Y, Boulieu R. Contribution of CYP3A4, CYP2B6, and CYP2C9 isoforms to N-demethylation of ketamine in human liver microsomes. Drug Metab Dispos. 2002;30(7):853–8.

218. Kimura Y, Ito H, Ohnishi R, Hatano T. Inhibitory effects of polyphenols on human cytochrome P450 3A4 and 2C9 activity. Food Chem Toxicol. 2010;48(1):429–35. doi:10.1016/j. fct.2009.10.041. S0278-6915(09)00502-X [pii].

219. Miners JO, Birkett DJ. Cytochrome P4502C9: an enzyme of major importance in human drug metabolism. Br J Clin Pharmacol. 1998;45(6):525–38.

220. Si D, Wang Y, Zhou YH, Guo Y, Wang J, Zhou H, Li ZS, Fawcett JP. Mechanism of CYP2C9 inhibition by flavones and flavonols. Drug Metab Dispos. 2009;37(3):629–34. doi:10.1124/ dmd.108.023416. dmd.108.023416 [pii].

221. He N, Zhang WQ, Shockley D, Edeki T. Inhibitory effects of H1-antihistamines on CYP2D6- and CYP2C9-mediated drug metabolic reactions in human liver microsomes. Eur J Clin Pharmacol. 2002;57(12):847–51.
222. Zhou SF, Xue CC, Yu XQ, Li C, Wang G. Clinically important drug interactions potentially involving mechanism-based inhibition of cytochrome P450 3A4 and the role of therapeutic drug monitoring. Ther Drug Monit. 2007;29(6):687–710. doi:10.1097/FTD.0b013e31815c16f5.
223. Feierman DE, Melinkov Z, Nanji AA. Induction of CYP3A by ethanol in multiple in vitro and in vivo models. Alcohol Clin Exp Res. 2003;27(6):981–8. doi:10.1097/01.ALC.0000071738.53337.F4.
224. Kumagai T, Suzuki H, Sasaki T, Sakaguchi S, Miyairi S, Yamazoe Y, Nagata K. Polycyclic aromatic hydrocarbons activate CYP3A4 gene transcription through human pregnane X receptor. Drug Metab Pharmacokinet. 2012;27(2):200–6.
225. Medina-Diaz IM, Arteaga-Illan G, de Leon MB, Cisneros B, Sierra-Santoyo A, Vega L, Gonzalez FJ, Elizondo G. Pregnane X receptor-dependent induction of the CYP3A4 gene by o, p'-1,1,1,-trichloro-2,2-bis (p-chlorophenyl)ethane. Drug Metab Dispos. 2007;35(1):95–102. doi:10.1124/dmd.106.011759.

Chapter 2
Aortitis

**Alessandro Della Corte, Marianna Buonocore,
and Ciro Bancone**

One Definition for Multiple Diseases: Classification, Epidemiology, Etiopathogenesis

"Aortitis" is a pathological term literally indicating inflammation of the aorta. It is used in nosography as a comprehensive term, encompassing the multiple etiologies possibly causing aortic wall inflammation [1]. A suggested classification of those etiologies distinguishes between two groups, i.e. infectious or non-infectious: within non-infectious aortitides, it discriminates different diseases following the current classification criteria for vasculitides (Table 2.1).

Infectious aortitis is a life-threatening disease, with high inherent risk of acute complications such as aortic aneurysm rupture; non-infectious forms however are often characterized by an indolent and insidious course, with progressive

———————
A. Della Corte, MD, PhD (✉) • C. Bancone
Cardiac Surgery Unit, Department of Cardiothoracic Sciences,
Monaldi Hospital, University of Naples II, Naples, Italy
e-mail: aledellacorte@libero.it

M. Buonocore
Cardiac Surgery School, Department of Cardiothoracic Sciences,
University of Naples II, Naples, Italy

A. Evangelista, C.A. Nienaber (eds.), *Pharmacotherapy
in Aortic Disease*, Current Cardiovascular Therapy, Vol. 7,
DOI 10.1007/978-3-319-09555-4_2,
© Springer International Publishing Switzerland 2015

TABLE 2.1 Classification of aortitis

Non-infectious[a]

Associated with vasculitides

  With large-vessel vasculitis

    Giant cell arteritis[b]

    Takayasu arteritis[b]

  With variable vessel vasculitis

    Cogan's syndrome[b]

    Behçet's disease[c]

  With medium- and small-vessel vasculitis

    Polyarteritis nodosa[d]

    Wegener arteritis[d]

    Microscopic polyangiitis[d]

Associated with systemic rheumatic disorders

  HLA-B27 associated spondyloarthropathies

    Ankylosing spondylitis[b]

    Reiter syndrome[c]

  Replapsing polychondritis[c]

  Systemic lupus erythematosus[d]

  Rheumatoid arthritis[d]

  Sarcoidosis[d]

"Single organ" vasculitis

  Isolated idiopathic aortitis (thoracic)

  Isolated idiopathic periaortitis (abdominal)

  Idiopathic retroperitoneal fibrosis (Ormond disease)

  Inflammatory abdominal aortic aneurysm

  Radiation-induced aortitis

(continued)

TABLE 2.1 (continued)

Infectious

Luetic (syphilis)

Mycobacterial (tubercolosis)

Bacterial

Salmonella spp.

Staphylococcus spp.

Streptococcus pneumonia

[a]Non-infective forms of aortitis (except radiation-induced aortitis) are here classified following the 2012 Chapel Hill Consensus Conference Classification of vasculitides [2]: "large-vessel", "medium-vessel" and "small-vessel" indicate the arteries preferentially involved; variable-vessel = large, medium and small arteries are evenly involved
[b]Vasculitis with common involvement of the aorta (>10 %)
[c]With less common involvement of the aorta (<10 %)
[d]Only case reports of aortic involvement or very small series reported

worsening, leading to significant quality-of-life limitations and potentially lethal evolutions. As a result of the different pathophysiological processes underlying the various forms of aortitis, it can in turn assume the phenotypes of dilative or obstructive disease of the aorta and its main branches, and present either isolated or within one of the several possible associated systemic syndromes, with or without involvement of other organs, eventually resulting in a myriad of diverse clinical pictures. A high index of diagnostic suspicion is necessary to avoid the complications and a correct differential diagnosis among the different etiologies is required to timely set the correct therapeutic strategy [1]. Diagnosis and differentiation can take advantage today of well-codified clinical criteria, at least for the most frequent forms of aortitis, multiple imaging modalities, laboratory tests and, to some extent, histology. In this chapter, we will address the description of aortitis and its treatment, emphasizing the above multiplicity of etiologies, involved mechanisms and clinical pictures, and focusing on the pharmacotherapy of the most common and notable forms of aortitis.

Non-infectious Aortitis

Non-infectious aortitis is more frequently encountered than infectious aortitis: inflammation is secondary to an autoimmune reaction in most of the non-infectious diseases, idiopathic in a minority of cases. The association between autoimmune ("rheumatic") diseases and aortic involvement is well known, but the prevalence of aortic involvement in the different rheumatic diseases is quite variable: in some of them, namely large-vessel vasculitides, aortic involvement is, by definition, part of the canonical clinical picture (e.g. Takayasu arteritis, giant cell arteritis); in others (e.g. spondyloarthropathies or anti-neutrophil cytoplasmic antibody-related diseases) an arterial inflammation, possibly but not regularly involving also the aorta, can be observed as a part of a systemic or multiorgan involvement. In fact, according to the 2012 Chapel Hill Consensus Conference Nomenclature [2], vasculitides that affect large arteries more often than the others are named "large-vessel vasculitis", those affecting predominantly medium caliber arteries are referred to as "medium-vessel vasculitis" and those affecting predominantly small size vessels are named "small-vessel vasculitis" (Table 2.1). Consistently, in 2006 a review on aortic involvement in rheumatic disorders listed Takayasu arteritis and giant cell arteritis among those most frequently affecting the aorta (>10 % patients), along with long-standing ankylosing spondylitis and Cogan syndrome; rheumatic diseases in which aortic involvement is an uncommon (<10 %) but well-documented complication include rheumatoid arthritis, sero-negative spondyloarthropathies, Behçet disease and relapsing polychondritis; rheumatic diseases with isolated case reports of aortic involvement or uncertain involvement include sarcoidosis, antineutrophil cytoplasmic antibody-associated aortitis (Wegener granulomatosis and *polyarteritis nodosa*), and systemic lupus eryhematosus [3].

Giant-cell arteritis (GCA), also known as Horton's (temporal) arteritis, is a chronic inflammatory large- and medium-vessel vasculitis that affects persons older than 50 years of age (reported male to female ratio ranges 1:2 to 2:3). GCA is much more common than Takayasu arteritis in the general population, with an estimated incidence of about 19 cases/million/year among patients over 50 years of age [4]. Although there is a markedly increased incidence of GCA in northern Europe and in populations with similar ethnic background [5], the disease can occur in all populations. The rate of aortic involvement in GCA is classically reported around 15–18 % (with a predominance of the ascending aorta, but possible involvement of the abdominal), however subclinical inflammation of the aorta may be present in a notably larger proportion of GCA patients. Branches most commonly involved are those arising from the external carotid artery, especially the superficial temporal artery, but ophthalmic, vertebral, coronary, and mesenteric arteries may also be involved.

The etiology of GCA is not well established. Polymorphisms of genes such as tumor necrosis factor-alpha (TNF-α), vascular endothelial growth factor (VEGF), endothelial nitric oxide synthase (eNOS), intercellular adhesion molecule (ICAM)-1, IL-6, and others appear to be more frequent in patients with GCA, although their pathogenetic role is still to be determined. It has been also postulated that a still unknown infectious pathogen may trigger the aberrant immune response [6].

The characteristic pathology feature of GCA is the presence of granulomatous inflammatory reaction in the vessel wall, with mostly macrophages, CD4$^+$ T-cells and giant multinucleated cells constituting the granulomas, particularly located at the intima-media border, but also B-cells. Giant cells can actually be absent in 30–40 % cases. The CD4$^+$ lymphocytes differentiate into T-helpers and produce interferon-gamma (IFN-γ), which activates macrophages, in turn producing reactive oxygen species and proteolytic enzymes, including matrix metalloproteases, the effectors of arterial wall elastic matrix degradation [7]. Lymphocytes and macrophages' products, including TNF-α and IL-6, also enter the blood and are responsible for the systemic clinical syndrome in GCA (see next section). Alternatively or adjunctively, a systemic inflammatory response may stimulate pattern recognition receptors at vascular level thereby activating vascular dendritic cells, in turn initiating T-cell response. The intima may be thickened and the medial elastic *laminae* fragmented, whereas in the late stages intimal changes may be minimal and medial changes are largely constituted by fibrosis.

Also known as pulseless disease or Martorell syndrome, Takayasu arteritis (TKA) is a necrotizing and obliterative segmental, large-vessel panarteritis of unknown cause with a predilection for young women (>80 % of cases). Epidemiology varies in the different geographic areas: in the United States, incidence estimates from Olmstead County, Minnesota, are 2.6 cases/million/year, whereas in Sweden and Germany they are 1–1.2 cases/million/year [8] Autopsy studies in Japan document a much higher prevalence, with evidence of TKA in 1 every 3,000 individuals. Also, the age of disease onset differs: it is earlier (15–25 years) in Asians compared to European women (40 years) [9]. Involvement of the aorta is frequent, reported between 80 and >90 %. The most commonly affected aortic segment is the abdominal aorta, however ascending aorta involvement has been described as more typical in Japanese women [3].

Although the exact etiology of TKA is not well known, a prior tubercular or streptococcal infection, genetic factors, and autoimmune mechanisms (possible association with rheumatoid arthritis) have been implicated as etiological factors [9]. The pathogenetic mechanisms are unknown as well, although it is considered to be antigen-driven cell-mediated autoimmune processes, although the specific antigenic stimuli have not been identified [10]. Vessel injury occurs as a result of invasion by leukocytes (including T-lymphocytes, NK-cells, B-lymphocytes, macrophages and others) deriving from the *vasa vasorum*, migrating to the intimal layer and producing a number of cytokines, including interleukin-6 (IL-6), tumor necrosis factor-alpha

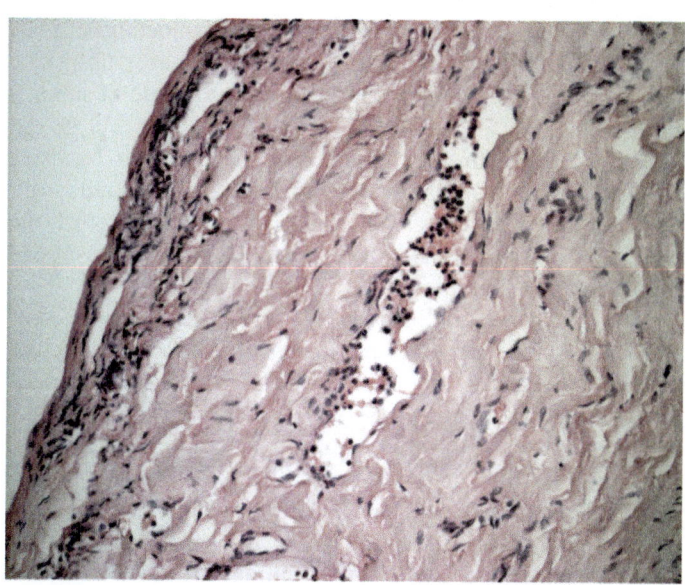

FIGURE 2.1 Histology findings of early stage non-infectious aortitis. Hematoxylin-eosin coloration shows multiple infiltrates of lymphocytes in the adventitia and sub-adventitial media, particularly surrounding the *vasa vasorum*, along with areas of initial focal medial elastic fibers disruption

(TNF-α), B-cell activating factor (BAFF) and others. Myointimal proliferation most commonly results, leading to stenosis of the vessel (most commonly the abdominal aorta) or its branches (especially supra-aortic vessels, iliac arteries and renal arteries), however medial smooth muscle cell necrosis and derangement of the extracellular matrix is another possible evolution, leading to aneurysm formation in 45 % cases (more common at the aortic root and ascending tract) [8]. Aside from the presence of granulomas, possibly including giant cells, in the aortic wall (particularly in the adventitia) and of perivascular cuffing of the *vasa vasorum*, histopathology usually reveals lymphoplasma-cytic infiltrate of adventitia and media (Fig. 2.1), a non-specific finding present in a number of rheumatic disorders, such as relapsing polychondritis, systemic lupus erythematosus (SLE), ankylosing spondylitis, as well as in aortitis of infectious or toxic etiology. At late stages (at least >5 years of disease), unspecific wall calcification is observed, especially in the case of stenotic evolution.

Indeed, the pathology pictures of the different forms of aortitis show substantial overlap, and contribute to make differential diagnosis quite challenging. In this perspective, the stenotic lesions, with thickened intima and media, have been reported as pathognomonic of TKA [8].

Ankylosing Spondylitis (AS) is an HLA-B27 disease classified as a seronegative spondyloarthritis, since it is not characterized by circulating rheumatoid factor. Risk of aortic involvement (predominantly aortic valve, root, ascending aorta) increases with disease duration. Pathology studies of the sacroiliac joints in patients with AS have shown a prominent role of synovitis and subchondral myxoid bone marrow changes, processes mediated by activated T-lymphocyte-derived TNF-α and TGF-β, in initiating intra-articular joint destruction; a *Klebsiella pneumoniae* infection may participate in providing an antigen that reaches the synovia and initiates T-cell responses in genetically susceptible individuals [11]. Similar mechanisms could induce the typical fibrosis changes of AS-associated valvulitis and aortitis: in particular at the level of the proximal aorta, *vasa vasorum* narrowing, fibrotic changes in the adventitia, medial matrix disruption and fibrosis and myointimal proliferation ensue [12].

Cogan's syndrome (CS) is a rare disease of young adults, with a mean age of 29 years at disease onset, defined by the presence of both ocular (keratitis) and inner ear inflammation [13]. Aortitis with valvulitis and aortic insufficiency has been documented as occurring from 2 weeks to 12 years after the initial diagnosis of the syndrome and has an estimated prevalence of up to 10 % [1, 3]. Etiopathogenesis is unknown: formerly believed to derive from a *Clamydia spp*. infection, today, after the finding of autoantibodies and lymphocyte activation against corneal and endothelial antigens, it is considered an autoimmune disorder [14]. Histologic analysis of the aortic wall reveals inflammation with prominent lymphocytic infiltration, destruction of medial elastic tissue, fibrosis, and neovascularization, which finally result in aneurysm formation [15].

Behçet disease (BD) is a rare, multisystemic, and chronic inflammatory disease of unknown etiology, characterized by mucocutaneous manifestations (aphtous ulcers), especially including genital and oral ulcers and often-severe sight-threatening inflammatory eye disease. It can be associated (up to 30–40 % cases) with vasculitic manifestations in arteries and veins of variable size [2]. The frequency of aortic involvement in BD varies according to different studies, ranging from 50 % of patients in reports from Turkey and Italy [16], to <1 % in other studies including only clinically significant aortic aneurysms [17]. Macroscopically, saccular aneurysms affecting the abdominal and/or thoracic aorta and their branches are typical of BD. Histopathology of the involved aorta shows lymphocytic infiltration mixed with histiocytes and eosinophils with giant cells around vasa vasorum of media and adventitia. Destruction of media leads to aneurysm formation and may proceed to pseudoaneurysm formation and rupture [18]. Aortitis derives not from direct large-vessel inflammation but rather due to vasculitis of the *vasa vasorum* that supply the vessel wall.

Apart from AS, other HLA-27-associated seronegative spondyloarthropathies can present with vascular involvement and potentially, but more rarely compared to the other abovementioned syndromes, with aortitis. These include Reiter's syndrome, an arthritic disease of the lower limbs associated with typical cutaneous lesions and relapsing polychondritis, affecting proteoglycan rich tissues, such as cartilages and vessels. Less frequently, some of the anti-neutrophil cytoplasmic antibody- (ANCA-) related diseases, namely Wegener's granulomatosis, microscopic polyangiitis and polyarteritis nodosa, which more typically involve small-size vessels, can be associated with large-vessel involvement and therefore aortitis. Whether aortitis in such cases is initiated by *vasa vasorum* involvement or by primitive inflammation of the intimal layer ("intimitis") has not been clarified yet [19].

Following the 2012 Chapell Hill Consensus Conference Nomenclature [2], isolated idiopathic aortitis (more frequently observed at the abdominal level) should be classified within the group of "single organ" vasculitides. Idiopathic aortitis is characterized by aortic wall inflammation in absence of any systemic disease or infection, and it usually involves the ascending aorta and arch. This condition affects women more often than men (3:2 ratio) and is asymptomatic until it is discovered incidentally or by post-surgical histological analysis [20]. In those latter cases, macroscopic appearance can already suggest inflammatory etiology, i.e. by the typical diffuse irregular scarring of the intima, referred to as "tree-barking" sign [1]. Histology can vary, however overlapping with the spectrum of lesions already mentioned above for specific etiologies. Infiltrates can include macrophages, T-cells, B-cells and also giant multinuclear cells. Idiopathic inflammatory aneurysms of the abdominal aorta, constituting 5–25 % of all abdominal aneurysms [21], are characterized by thickening of the aortic wall, associated with a considerable peri-aortic reaction and dense adhesions. They are more frequently observed in young males with familiar history of aneurysm, and use of tobacco smoke. Retroperitoneal fibrosis is characterized by a chronic inflammation with fibrous tissue deposition in the retroperitoneum surrounding the aorta, the stem of its main abdominal branches and the ureters. Complications include hydronephrosis, aortic-enteric fistula, and secondary bacterial infections [1].

It has been recently discovered that some cases of idiopathic aortitis, idiopathic aneurysm and retroperitoneal fibrosis are actually secondary to a so-called "IgG4-related systemic disease", in which multiple organs are involved by inflammatory infiltrates constituted by IgG4-expressing plasmacells, and abnormally high levels of IgG4 are found in the serum. This syndrome was first described in patients with autoimmune forms of pancreatitis, but other glands (e.g. salivary glands and thyroid) can be involved, as well as lungs, kidneys, heart, retroperitoneum, mediastinum and aorta [22].

Infectious Aortitis

Infectious aortitis is an infectious and inflammatory process of the aortic wall directly induced by micro-organisms. In the preantibiotic era, it was most likely a complication of bacterial endocarditis secondary to *Streptococcus pyogenes*, *Streptococcus pneumoniae*, and *Staphylococcus*. Nowadays, the most common pathogens, which account for almost 40 % of infections, include *Staphylococcus aureus* and *Salmonella spp*. Other pathogens involved include *Treponema pallidum*, *Mycobacterium tuberculosis* (less common today in developed countries), and other bacteria such as *Listeria*, *Bacteroides fragilis*, *Clostridium septicum*, and *Campylobacter jejuni* [23]. The aorta is normally very resistant to infection; however, an abnormal aortic wall, like that associated with atherosclerotic disease, preexisting aneurysm, medial degeneration, diabetes, vascular/valvular malformation, medical devices, or surgery, makes it more susceptible to infection, if a bacteriaemia occurs [24]. Mechanisms of infection include hematogenous spread (e.g. in non-typhoid *Salmonella spp.* Gastroenteritis), contiguous seeding from adjacent infection, septic emboli of the aortic *vasa vasorum* and traumatic or iatrogenic inoculation. Infected (or "mycotic") aortic aneurysms are part of the spectrum of infectious aortitis and account for <3 % cases of aortic aneurysms. Men are affected more often than women, with most cases seen in adults after the fifth decade of life: elderly or immunocompromised patients are more susceptible to bacterial seeding at the level of preexisting aortic lesions. Both host leukocytes and responsible bacteria can induce aortic wall lesions, namely extracellular matrix degradation, by producing a variety of proteases including matrix metalloprotease-1, −2, −8 and −9 [25]. The collagenase activity may be relatively localized, leading to formation of a saccular abdominal aortic aneurysm or pseudoaneurysm in an otherwise normal appearing vessel. Collagenase activity may also be intensive, which may explain the rapid course associated with infected abdominal aortic aneurysms. Typical pathology findings include aortic atherosclerosis, acute suppurative inflammation, neutrophil infiltration, and bacterial clumps. About two-thirds of patients can show acute inflammation superimposed on severe chronic atherosclerosis; the remainder show atherosclerosis with chronic inflammation or pseudoaneurysms [25].

A Challenging Diagnosis

Clinical Pictures

Since symptoms and signs associated with aortitis during the initial phase of the disease are unspecific, a high level of diagnostic suspicion is required for an early diagnosis and a timely treatment.

Giant cell arteritis usually develops later in life compared to TKA, with only few cases reported at an age younger than 50, and is twice more frequent in women than in men. The clinical onset is quite abrupt so that patients are often able to tell a certain date for the appearance of symptoms. The frequent involvement of the temporal artery leads to the most evident symptoms, i.e. localized headache, scalp tenderness, jaw claudication. Either in association with those symptoms or isolately, the involvement of other vessels, also including the aorta, may cause impairment of vision (anterior ischemic optic neuropathy, *amaurosis fugax* or diplopia) together with signs of inflammation, fever of unknown origin with night sweats, claudication of the upper limbs, rarely hearing impairment and dizziness, stroke, symptoms of aortic insufficiency and myocardial ischemia [26].

Clinical examination evidences alterations of the temporal artery region, which appears tender, swollen, firm, beaded or reddened with a reduction of the artery pulse. Similar signs can be found in the occipital region as well. At the level of the upper limbs there may be an asymmetry of radial pulses and blood pressure or bruits of the subclavian and axillary region. Symptoms and signs of an associated *polymyalgia reumatica* can also be present, including reduced range of motion of shoulders, particularly with impaired arm abduction, a reduced internal and external rotation of the hip, tenderness of the upper arms and thighs. When the suspicion of GCA arise, fundoscopy by an experienced investigator may be appropriate, even in patients showing no eye impairment [26].

The diagnosis of GCA relies on clinical, laboratory, and histological criteria as described in the 1990 American College of Rheumatology classification scheme [27] (Table 2.3).

The existence of an atypical pattern of GCA has been described, in which the temporal artery is spared and the disease more consistently affects large arteries, such as aorta. In this case the clinical scenario may be completely different, mostly dominated by systemic symptoms as fever, decline in general wellbeing, laboratory evidence of inflammation and rarely pain in the lower back or abdomen. This makes reaching the clinical diagnosis of GCA with large vessel involvement even later that for temporal arteritis, sometimes only after histology of the intraoperative specimen [28].

Early published data on aortic involvement in patients with GCA were based on the rate of aortic aneurysms diagnosed fortuitously or after acute events (aortic dissection and rupture of an aortic aneurysm). Thus, in retrospective studies, the prevalence of aortitis ranged from 3 to 18 % [29]. Owing to the introduction of new imaging techniques, capable to show aortic involvement before the development of structural abnormalities, rates of aortic involvement ranging between 33 and 45 % have been disclosed.

Aortic involvement is most often localized at the ascending aorta, and occurs quite late during the natural history of GCA (median time from diagnosis 11 years for the thoracic location) most often manifesting as annuloaortic ectasia, determining aortic valve insufficiency or ascending aortic aneurysm. Acute aortic dissection is a possible complication and occasionally represents the first evidence of disease (within 1 year median time of diagnosis). Abdominal aortic aneurysm can also develop and aneurysms are usually present in the thoracic descending segment in the late phase of the disease [30].

Diagnosis of *Takayasu arteritis* is usually delayed, as a result of the vague nature of the symptoms in its initial phase (often referred to as "pre-pulseless phase"). Mirroring the general systemic inflammation, symptoms of this stage may include fever, malaise, weight loss, night sweat, arthralgia and myalgia [31]. In the late phase the chronic inflammatory process leads to vascular lesions such as aneurismal dilatation, as a consequence of disruption of the connective scaffold in the arterial wall. During the late ("pulseless") phase, systemic manifestations usually remit significantly and symptoms are mainly related to organ ischemia: arm claudication, dizziness, headache, stroke, visual impairment, renal arterial hypertension, angina, myocardial infarction, pulmonary hypertension [26].

The involvement of the aorta and its main branches is common in this disease, most frequently in the abdominal segment, followed by the descending thoracic aorta and the aortic arch. A 53 % prevalence of aorta stenosis has been reported, in 70 % cases affecting the abdominal aorta [32]. Rapid expansion of aortic aneurysms (45 % cases), aortic rupture (33 %) and (more rarely) intramural hematoma and acute aortic dissection, constitute possible severe complications reported to occur in TKA aortitis [33, 34].

Clinical examination should focus on vascular and neurologic systems: a check of the arterial pulses and auscultation of the subclavian, carotid, abdominal and femoral region may evidence asymmetry of pulses and bruits; a bilateral check of blood pressure in the arms and in the legs should always be performed, as it may show significant pressure differences; a neurological examination may detect signs of an ischemic neurological damage [26].

The onset of specific symptoms and signs of TKA is usually early, i.e. during the third or fourth decade of life. Classification criteria have been developed in 1990 by the American College of Rheumatology for TKA [35] (Table 2.2). The most recently issued classification of TKA, based on the vessels involved, distinguishes: type I, involvement of the main branches from the aortic arch; type IIa, involvement of the ascending aorta, aortic arch and its branches; type IIb,

TABLE 2.2 Diagnostic criteria for Takayasu's arteritis (according to the American College of Rheumatology)

Age of 40 years or less at disease onset

Claudication of the extremities

Decreased pulsation at one or both brachial arteries (compared to pulses at lower limbs)

Systolic blood pressure difference of >10 mmHg between the two arms

Bruit over the subclavean artery or the aorta

Angiography evidence of focal or segmental occlusion or narrowing of large arteries (including the aorta), not resulting from arteriosclerosis or fibromuscular dysplasia

If at least three criteria are present, the diagnosis is made, with sensitivity and specificity of 90 and 98 % respectively

involvement of the ascending aorta, aortic arch and its branches, and thoracic descending aorta; type III, involvement of the thoracic descending aorta, abdominal aorta and/or renal arteries; type IV, involvement of the abdominal aorta and/or renal arteries; and type V, the combined features of type IIb and IV [8].

Non infectious aortitis may be secondary to rheumatic disease, usually driven by aberrant immune responses, giving rise to clinical pictures in which the specific manifestations of the aortic involvement may be confounded by the systemic clinical scenario dominated by the underlying disease or may initially be overlooked by both patients and physicians.

Ankylosing spondylitis (AS) is part of a group of diseases called spondyloarthropaties, associated with HLA-B27 antigen, characterized by sacroilitis, enthesitis, inflammatory bowel disease or psoriasis. It begins with back pain and stiffness during the second or third decade of life, affecting men two to three times more than women. Diagnosis requires at least four of the following criteria: age younger than 40 at onset, insidious onset of arthropathy, back pain for more than 3 months, morning stiffness, improvement with exercise.

Aortitis is present in 80 % of patients with long-standing AS, usually affecting the aortic root and the aortic valve, with insufficiency. AS may also affect the myocardium with impairment of the conduction system [36].

Cogan's syndrome is a rare disease, characterized by ocular, inner ear, and vascular inflammation. Cardiovascular manifestations include aortitis and necrotizing vasculitis, which may induce coronary, renal, and iliac artery stenosis. About 10 % of patients may have aortitis with aortic aneurysm, and valvulitis with aortic insufficiency. Young male patients are predominantly affected, usually presenting with eye redness, photophobia, or eye pain from interstitial keratitis, audiovestibular manifestations similar to those in Ménière syndrome, neural deafness, and possibly symptoms of aortic insufficiency with or without associated ischemic syndromes due to coronary or iliac stenosis, or hypertension related to renal artery stenosis [37].

Relapsing polychondritis is a paroxysmal and progressive inflammatory disease of the cartilaginous structures, affecting the ear, nose, and hyaline cartilage of the tracheobronchial tree. It is caused by autoimmune response against proteoglycan rich tissues. Aortic involvement may be observed in 5 % of patients, resulting in aneurysm formation in the thoracic and abdominal aorta and obliterans vasculitis in other medium-sized and large arteries. Typical of the acute phases is the histological picture of vasa vasorum extending also through both the media and the edematous intima [38].

Aortitis may be associated also with *Behçet's disease*, a systemic chronic disease with typically relapsing course affecting predominantly males of the Mediterranean area and Eastern countries. Its diagnosis is made upon the criteria established by the International Study Group for Behçet's Disease: presence of oral ulceration and at least two between genital ulceration, eye lesions, skin lesions or a positive pathergy test. In one-fifth of patients affected by aortitic complication, multiple pseudoaneurysms can develop, also involving the iliac, femoral, popliteal, and subclavian arteries.

Less frequently, aortitis may be associated with other rheumatologic diseases including rheumatoid arthritis (5 %), Reiter disease (<1 %) and systemic lupus erythematosus (few cases reported).

No specific clinical picture is associated with *idiopathic aortitis* of the thoracic segment, which can indeed be asymptomatic and detected incidentally: diagnosis is made in such cases at the time of histopathology review after thoracic aortic aneurysm surgery. In some cases unspecific thoracic pain can occur, but in most instances no systemic inflammatory symptoms are present. An idiopathic inflammatory aneurysm of the abdominal aorta can present with back or abdominal pain and constitutional symptoms, similarly to other non-infectious etiologies, and differentiation can be suggested by laboratory results and by histological analysis after surgical excision. Clinical onset of retroperitoneal fibrosis can be accompanied by renal function impairment, due to ureteral obstruction and in some cases by intestinal symptoms (e.g. abdominal pain and/or mass with or without sickness and vomit, related to duodenal obstruction) [39].

Infectious aortitis is a severe clinical entity, insidious insofar as it can be virtually undistinguished from non-infectious forms in terms of clinical presentation, and associated with a high inherent risk of acute and life-threatening complications. *Salmonella spp.* are reported to be the commonest pathogens involved in infective aortitis, accounting for almost 40 % of infective aortitis together with *Staphylococcus aureus*, mostly involving the abdominal aorta. The more frequent route of infection is a bacteremia following an ingestion of contaminated food, and a subsequent colonization of a pre-existing aortic atherosclerotic lesion. Aortic infection from a contiguous site, such as a paravertebral abscess complicating a spondylodiscitis is less common. Rare complications are aorto-enteric fistula and endo-myocardial abscess. The natural history of infectious aortitis is characterized by the progressive expansion of the aneurysm, with a greater tendency to rupture, compared to other etiologies, if not diagnosed and treated promptly. The majority of patients affected by infective aortitis are symptomatic, especially in the aneurysmal stage of the disease. Fever and back pain are the most common symptoms, being present respectively in the 77 % and 65 % of patients with infected aortic aneurysm. Chills, sweats, abdominal symptoms as nausea and vomiting are other possible symptoms [40].

Pneumoccoccal aortitis is rare and is usually due to bacteriemic spread from distant infection foci, such as pneumonia, urinary tract infections, endocarditis, osteomyelitis, cellulitis. Abdominal aorta is the segment most often involved by pneumococcal aortitis, followed by descending thoracic aorta [41].

Aortitis may be a clinical consequence of *Treponema pallidum* determining obliterative vasculitis of aortic *vasa vasorum*, during the third (late) phase of syphilis. After a progressive decrease in its epidemiological importance over the last century, primary syphilis has doubled its incidence during the first decade of the new century, with a majority of cases among homosexual men. This probably heralds a new resurgence of tertiary syphilis, in the next years, with a new epidemiological pattern of infective aortitis. Luetic aortitis typically involves the tubular portion of the ascending aorta, aortic arch and descending thoracic aorta, sparing the sinuses of Valsalva. Consequently, aortic insufficiency associated to aortic root dilatation has been only seldom reported. Clinical diagnosis is most often made based upon serologic confirmation of syphilis and a characteristic pattern of vascular involvement [42].

Other microorganisms, such as *Enterococcus spp.*, *Listeria monocytogenes*, *Bacteroides fragilis*, *Clostridium septicum*, human immunodeficiency virus (HIV), *Mycobacterium tuberculosis* may less frequently cause infectious aortitis. A positive history for signs and symptoms of the primary infection should guide the diagnosis towards infectious etiology, if an aortitis has been detected, importantly distinguishing it from autoimmune etiology. The warning has been issued that tuberculous aortitis, possibly evolving towards vessel stenosis or occlusion, might be misdiagnosed as Takayasu arteritis and erroneously treated by glucocorticoids, which may obviously worsen the infection course.

Imaging and Laboratory

The relevant, though complementary role played by imaging in the diagnosis of aortitis was officially recognized in the 2010 American College of Cardiology / American Heart Association Guidelines for the diagnosis and management of patients with thoracic aortic disease (Class I, level C), as it was in the American College of Rheumatology criteria for the diagnosis of Takayasu arteritis [35, 43].

Imaging provides important information for establishing the diagnosis, contributing in the differentiation between aortitis and other causes of aortic dilatation or large vessel stenosis, estimating the extent of disease, helping to monitor disease activity and response to therapy, and guiding biopsies (in GCA-associated temporal arteritis). The different available imaging methods are used to describe, with different specificity, the two elements of (1) the aortic lumen and (2) aortic wall changes. In large-vessel vasculitis, imaging studies document the anatomic distribution of the lesion, characterized by homogeneous artery wall swelling and aortic dilatation or peculiar large vessel stenoses with smoothly tapered luminal narrowing.

Giant cell arteritis typically involves the branches of the external carotid arteries. The aorta and its main branches are usually unaffected but the possible occurrence of an atypical pattern of large-vessel GCA with negative temporal artery biopsy is reported in up to 25 % of patients [26] and often unsuspected until life-threatening complications occur. Large-vessel form of GCA usually involves the axillary arteries bilaterally and less frequently the subclavian, brachial, femoro-popliteal axis or the aorta itself. However, because aortitis-related complications may be a source of both severe morbidity and mortality, routine screening for aortic involvement is mandatory in patients with any form of GCA [28].

The peripheral aortic branches are easily accessible to ultrasonography (US) that shows a perivascular hypoechoic halo similar to the finding at the temporal artery (the "halo sign"), which reflects wall edema. Soon after pharmacologic treatment initiation, wall edema decreases and US reveals an increase of the wall echogenicity because fibrosis occurs, being still visible in more than a half of patients even after 1 year of treatment [44]. When GCA affects arteries in the lower limbs, special attention must be paid for a differential diagnosis with atherosclerosis that often occurs at these sites but with different characteristics (atherosclerotic plaques are usually calcified, asymmetric and inhomogeneous) [45].

Computed tomography (CT) angiography is commonly the initial imaging study performed because it is diffusely available. It has an excellent spatial resolution and multidetector scanners allow multiplanar reformation and three-dimensional reconstruction. Actually, CT is less sensitive than other techniques, as magnetic resonance imaging (MRI) or positron-emission tomography (PET), for identifying early wall changes but in an advanced phase it is useful to reveal luminal changes such as stenosis, occlusion, dilatation, aneurysm, calcification and mural thrombi. Contrast-enhanced CT scan may help diagnosis of aortitis showing a concentric thickening (>3 mm) of the arterial wall with post-contrast enhancement [28].

MRI can provide accurate information on involvement of the aorta and its branches, moreover high resolution MRI can investigate temporal arteries. MRI is able to detect the earliest vascular inflammation in the vessel wall and also the luminal changes of the mature phase: findings in GCA include circumferential thickening of the vessel-wall in T1-weighted images, producing a high signal on T2-weighted images (wall edema), and post-gadolinium enhancement in the affected segment [28].

18-Fluorodeoxyglucose (18FDG) – PET-CT is a useful imaging modality in the assessment of active inflammation in

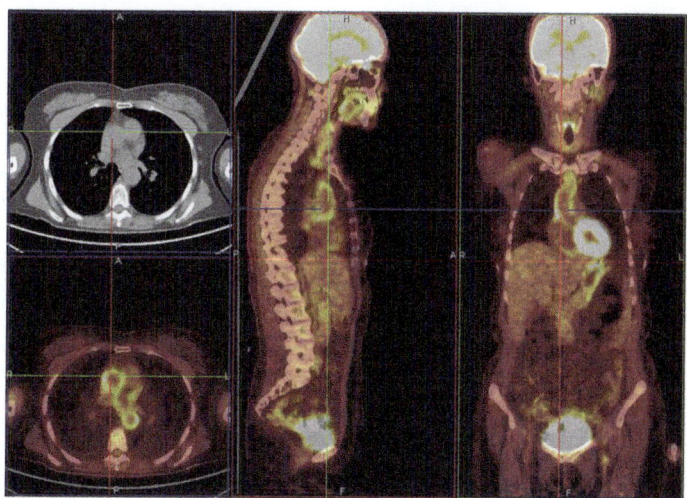

FIGURE 2.2 18FDG-PET-CT showing hyper-uptake at the level of the ascending aorta. Such levels of uptake are highly indicative of aortitis; lower levels may be associated with atherosclerotic lesions, whereas the normal has no detectable uptake (Courtesy of Drs M. Bifulco and F. Porcaro, Nuclear Medicine Diagnostics Unit of the Monaldi Hospital, Naples, Italy)

cardiovascular diseases including aortitis, atherosclerosis and acute dissection. Normally there is no radiotracer accumulation in the arterial wall, thus any 18FDG up-take can be consider a sign of inflammatory infiltrates or infection (Fig. 2.2). Large-vessel FDG uptake is usually graded on a 4-point scale: none (grade 0), lower than liver uptake (grade 1), similar to liver uptake (grade 2) and higher than liver uptake (grade 3). Grades 2–3 are relatively specific for vasculitis, while grade 1, or rarely 2, has been observed in atherosclerotic vessels [46]. Moreover, to exclude false positivity due to atherosclerosis (especially in lower limb lesions), some authors suggest relying only on the upper-body sites of 18-FDG uptake for the diagnosis of GCA [47]. In GCA 18FDG-PET may reveal early inflammation sites even in the absence of detectable structural changes at CT: abnormal uptake in the aortic arch or large thoracic arteries is found in more than 50 % of affected patients. This is of particular importance for establishing the diagnosis in atypical clinical scenarios with predominance of systemic signs of inflammation, with negative temporal artery biopsy [28]. Since inflammatory cell infiltration is likely to happen prior to the development of wall edema, PET can be even more sensitive for early aortitis than MRI. Contrary to MRI, PET cannot investigate cranial arteries because of its low spatial resolution and the background noise derived from the brain (high FDG uptake of the neuronal cells). PET may also be useful for monitoring the response to treatment: the persistence of 18FDG uptake in the arterial wall at follow-up despite an adequate therapy has been described to have a predictive role for vascular remodeling and aneurismal dilatation [48].

No specific laboratory tests exist for the diagnosis of GCA. Erythrocyte Sedimentation Rate (ESR) and also C Reactive Protein (CRP) readings are high in most patients, and ESR elevation is included between the diagnostic criteria, although up to 10 % of patients with documented GCA have normal sedimentation rates at the time of diagnosis. On the contrary, an elevated ESR can be seen in most of the disorders usually considered in the differential diagnosis of patients with possible vasculitis, notably infections and malignancies, thus limiting the diagnostic usefulness of this test. Acute phase reactants may serve as simple tools for monitoring disease activity during therapy. Many patients have mild to moderate anemia, thrombocytosis and slightly elevated transaminases [26, 43].

While large vessel GCA typically involves the axillary arteries, in *Takayasu's arteritis* the most commonly involved sites are the subclavian arteries (93 %), followed by the aorta (65 %), and the common carotid arteries (58 %) [26]. Other possible sites described for TKA are renal, vertebral, innominate, axillary, superior mesenteric, common iliac, and pulmonary arteries.

Differently from GCA, CT angiography is essential in the early steps of the diagnostic process for TKA, being the imaging technique with the highest predictive power for demonstrating the abnormalities of the affected vessels. The typical finding in the early stage of the disease is the wall thickening that has been described as the "double ring" sign. This is due to edema in the intimal layer which gives a low-density signal next to a high-density signal from the infiltrated media and adventitia. In the chronic phase of the disease (≥5 years) CT scan may show calcifications of the previous inflamed sites: these are commonly linear and tend to spare the ascending aorta [21].

MRI may also help in the diagnosis of TKA because of its intrinsic ability to investigate the early wall changes occurring before lumen stenosis develops, with findings similar to those in large-vessel GCA. Phase-contrast (PC) – MRI and magnetic resonance angiography (MRA) can also document multiple stenoses, mural thrombi, thickening of aortic valve cusps, and pericardial effusions [21, 49]. For the absence of ionizing radiations, MRI is recommended for serial imaging follow-up especially in young patients.

In a normal carotid wall, US shows an hypoechoic space known as the intima-media complex (IMC), in between two hyperechogenic layers. When edema occurs in the arterial wall, there is an increased and diffuse thickening of the IMC that has been referred to as "macaroni sign", unique of TKA [50]. This diffuse thickening, together with the arterial segments involved, help to differentiate vasculitis from atherosclerosis. The stenosing lesions evolve quite slowly, which explains the common presence of collaterals, with reported cases of reverse flow in vertebral arteries with or without the subclavian steal phenomenon in patients with Takayasu disease [51]. US is useful in TKA also for the investigation of the aortic valve, ascending aorta and pulmonary artery [52].

18FDG-PET represents a promising, yet not definitively established, method to help in the diagnosis of TKA in patients with constitutional symptoms and fever of unknown origin. Hybrid imaging with 18FDG-PET (detecting circumferential increased metabolic activity) and CT or MRI (allowing more precise anatomic localization of the disease) has emerged as a valuable tool in diagnosing and monitoring treatment response in TKA aortitis. The European League Against Rheumatism (EULAR) recommends PET, together with MRI, for diagnosing large-vessel vasculitis, most notably in patients with TKA, as histological documentation is difficult to obtain in the large-vessel forms of the disease [53].

In TKA laboratory test findings are similar to those of GCA. The ESR and CRP are in most cases highly elevated in active disease, although a smaller number of patients have normal ESR or CRP values [26].

When non-infectious aortitis is ascertained, in the absence of an identifiable vasculitis or rheumatic systemic syndrome with possible secondary aortic involvement, *idiopathic aortitis* is diagnosed. Usually the diagnosis is made post-operatively on the basis of the histological findings on the aortic specimen (giant cells or lymphoplasmacytic inflammation). Patients with idiopathic aortitis have more diffuse and more often extensive (also thoracic descending and thoraco-abdominal) dilatation of the aorta compared with those with non-inflammatory dilatations [54]. Idiopathic aortitis patients are generally older at presentation and have greater diameters than those with large vessel vasculitis-associated aortitis, probably related to the silently progressing nature of the disease [55]. CT-scan identifies the inflammatory aneurysm as a hypo-dense mass with thickening of the periaortic tissues that show delayed contrast enhancement in CT angiography following the rapid intra-luminal enhancement.

In idiopathic inflammatory abdominal aneurysms the thickening of the aortic wall/periaortic tissues typically spares the posterior aspect of the vessel [56]. CT is also important to asses possible adhesions of the mass with the abdominal organs in order to plan the surgical strategy (i.e. transperitoneal versus retroperitoneal approach). In the pre-operative phase, MRI helps detailing aneurysm localization (suprarenal versus infrarenal) and demonstrates the presence of periaortic inflammation, adventitial thickening and turbulent flow inside the aneurysm. Diffusion-weighted MR imaging shows a hyperintense halo surrounding the aneurysm.

FDG-PET helps to evaluate the grade of inflammation and also the extent of adhesions if combined to CT/MRI. US shows a periaortic hypoechoic mass that represents the inflammatory process surrounding a thickened aortic wall.

On CT-scan *retroperitoneal fibrosis* appears as a retroperitoneal paraspinal mass with soft-tissue density (isoattenuating compared to adjacent ileo-psoas muscles), surrounding the abdominal aorta and often encircling the ureters and the inferior vena cava, with a variable involvement of the abdominal organs including duodenum and pancreas. Usually this mass is not displacing the aorta form the anterior surface of the spine [57].

Clinical diagnosis of *infectious aortitis* is not simple given the unspecific nature of signs and symptoms, that are usually more evident only in an advanced stages of the disease (aneurysm expansion) or when acute complications occur (rupture of the aneurysm). The definitive etiology is determined only by blood cultures, which can be positive in 50–80 % of the patients, but imaging supports clinical examination and concur to discriminate among alternative diagnoses [57].

Contrast-enhanced CT is the imaging modality of choice in most medical centers because of its widespread availability and multiplanar capability. The association of imaging evidence of a saccular aortic aneurysm, positive blood cultures and typical symptoms of the original infectious focus is diagnostic of the full-blown clinical picture of infective aortitis. In the early stage, aneurysm may not be present but other signs can be evident, including aortic wall thickening with or without contrast enhancement, periaortic nodularity, periaortic soft tissue mass, fluid collections, fat stranding, increasing aortic diameters, and air within the aortic wall. Fluid collection and gas bubbles within the periaortic tissue are signs of impending rupture even in absence of an aneurysm. CT scan helps to discriminate alternative diagnoses such as intramural hematoma, aortic dissection, penetrating aortic ulcer, pseudoaneurysm [1]. MRI with gadolinium contrast can obtain a better imaging definition of earlier alterations of the aortic wall. Segments affected may appear thickened, enhanced and edematous in the edema-weighted sequences [58]. PET-CT can be a useful adjunct in infectious aortitis, depicting the activity phase of the infectious process.

A strict association between infective aortitis (particularly of the ascending tract) and infective valve endocarditis has been reported, especially in the pre-antibiotic era. Transoesophageal echocardiography is the gold standard method in the diagnosis of infective valve endocarditis, and at the same time it allows for thorough investigation of the proximal tract of the aorta to rule out signs of aortitis [59].

Without appropriate treatment, natural progression of infectious aortitis is rapid with the development of mycotic aneurysms and high propensity to rupture. The term mycotic aortic aneurysm was coined by Wilson in 1984 to describe an aneurysm developed on a previous unaffected aorta following an infective embolus originating from a valve endocarditis [60]; today it encompasses all aneurysms that develop as a complication of infective aortitis. Its incidence is rare, representing only 0.7–2.6 % of all aortic aneurysms, most frequently localized at the abdominal segment, followed by the descending thoracic aorta [61, 62]. At CT/MRI, a mycotic aneurysm (Fig. 2.3) appears as a saccular aneurysm with lobulated contours and possible additional features as periaortic soft tissue density mass, edema, fat stranding, and/or fluid collections. Rapid increase in size and/or change in shape of an aneurysm should increase the diagnostic suspicion for an infectious etiology [63].

Typically Enterococcus infections cause thoracic aortitis, whereas Salmonella spp. mostly affect the abdominal aorta, like in the pneumococcal aortitis [64]. Tubercular aortitis normally involves the aortic arch and the descending thoracic aorta as a focal pseudo-aneurysm with multiple out-pouching and wall thickening. This kind of lesion can be combined with caseous necrosis of periaortic lymph nodes, bones or paraspinal abscesses from which the infection has extended to the aorta for contiguity [65]. In the third phase of syphilis, cardiovascular system may be affected with manifestations as luetic aortitis, aortic aneurysm, aortic valvulitis with regurgitation

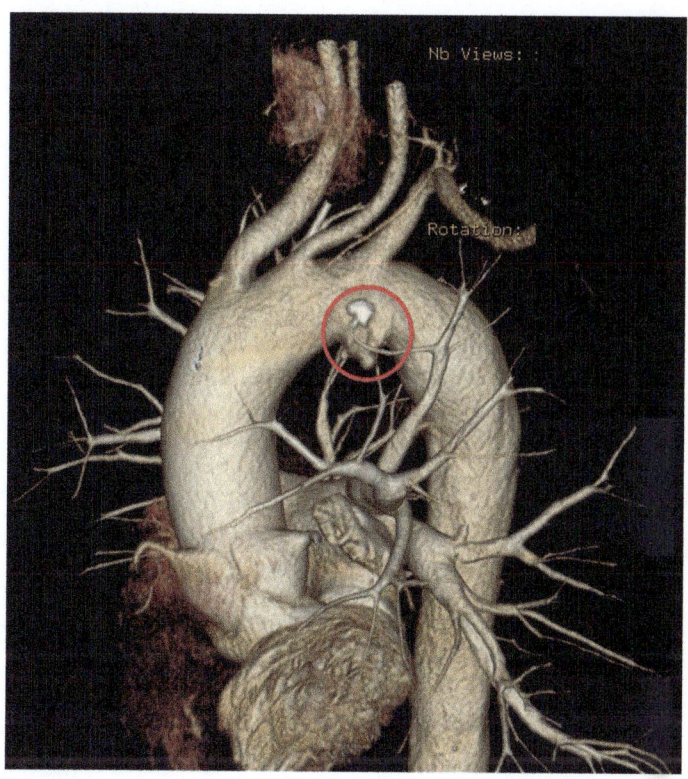

FIGURE 2.3 Multi-slice CT scan reconstruction in a patient with mycotic aneurysm of the aortic arch (*encircled in red*). The typical appearance of a small saccular aneurysm due to infectious aortitis (from *Escherichia spp.* in this patient) is evidenced, with its irregular profile due to multiple out-pouches. Location of the lesion is also typical, i.e. opposite the origin of aortic branches

and coronary stenosis. The most commonly involved site is the ascending aorta, followed by aortic arch and descending thoracic aorta. The infectious process normally evolves in aneurysmal disease with diffuse wall thickening and typical "tree-barking" appearance of the luminal surface at gross examination. On delayed enhancement CT scan the affected aortic wall may have a double-ring appearance mimicking Takayasu aortitis [66]. Giant syphilitic aneurysms involving the thoracic aorta and determining sternum erosion or rightward displacement of the mediastinum have been described [67, 68].

As for non-infectious aortitis, laboratory tests are complementary to imaging in the diagnosis of infectious aortitis. Leukocytosis and neutrophilia are present in 65–83 % of cases. ESR and CRP are elevated in most of the patients. Microbiology is of paramount importance to identify etiology in infectious aortitis. Blood cultures are positive in 50–85 % of the patients and a microorganism can be isolated from the excised aortic tissue in up to 76 % of the patients [24]. The diagnosis of syphilitic aortitis has to be confirmed by serologic tests. Serology include sensitive non-treponemal serologic tests (rapid plasma reagin test, Venereal Disease Research Laboratory test) and specific treponemal serologic tests (fluorescent treponemal antibody-absorption test, microhemagglutination-T pallidum test).

The Role of Pharmacotherapy in Aortitis

First-Line Pharmacotherapy of Non-infectious Aortitis

The vast majority of non-infectious forms of aortitis is represented by auto-immune disorders, namely vasculitis (e.g. GCA and TKA) and systemic diseases (e.g. Rheumatoid Arthritis and SA). Therefore, the mainstay of the pharmacotherapy for non-infectious aortitis is immunosuppressive therapy. While guidelines and official professional societies recommendations have been issued for the most epidemiologically relevant large-vessel vasculitides (although with quite low levels of supporting evidence) [53, 69], no specific pharmacologic protocols exist for the aortitis that occurs with variable frequencies in patients affected by vasculitides.

Glucocorticoids are the cornerstone of drug therapy for large-vessel vasculitides. Given the inherent risks of severe morbidities (e.g. ocular impairment in GCA, renal or coronary stenosis in TKA, etc.), a timely diagnosis, preferably before the onset of such organ complications, is crucial, so that glucocorticoids can be administered early and at high initial doses. According to the EULAR (European League Against Rheumatism) 2009 recommendations, the initial dose of prednisolone is 1 mg/kg/day, with a maximum dose of 60 mg/day, maintained for a month and tapered gradually, avoiding alternate day tapering, as it is associated with higher risk of relapses [53].

In Giant Cell Arteritis, according to the British Society of Rheumatology and British Health Professionals in Rheumatology guidelines, the sole clinical suspicion, even in the absence of histological confirmation on temporal artery biopsies, must prompt glucocorticoid therapy initiation [69] (Fig. 2.4). The starting protocol depends on the clinical picture at the time of diagnosis (stage of disease):

- Uncomplicated GCA (with no jaw claudication or visual disturbance): 40–60 mg prednisolone daily;
- Complicated GCA with evolving visual loss or *amaurosis fugax*: 500 mg to 1 g of i.v. methylprednisolone for 3 days before oral glucocorticoids;
- Complicated GCA with established visual loss: 60 mg prednisolone daily to protect the contralateral eye.

Patients often report a rapid response to therapy initiation, with early (hours or few days) recovery especially from systemic symptoms (malaise, fever, headache and polymyalgia), then from laboratory markers of early phase inflammation. Symptoms related to ischemic consequences of arterial stenosis may take more days or weeks to relieve (jaw claudication, temporary visual impairments, arm claudication). Temporal artery biopsy can remain positive for up to 6 weeks after treatment commencement. On the other hand, histological negativity should not exclude diagnosis of GCA in the presence of other three criteria (Table 2.3), whereas lack of rapid response to therapy in terms of systemic inflammation signs should induce to reconsideration of the diagnosis

Table 2.3 Diagnostic criteria for giant cell arteritis (according to the American College of Rheumatology)

Age of 50 years or more at disease onset
New localized headache
Temporal artery abnormalities to palpation (tenderness or decreased pulsation)
Erythrocyte sedimentation rate >50 mm/h
Mononuclear cell infiltration or granulomatous inflammation with or without giant cells in arterial biopsy

If at least three criteria are present, the diagnosis is made, with sensitivity and specificity of 94 and 91 % respectively

(Fig. 2.4). Only after disappearance of clinical symptoms, generally after at least 3–4 weeks, gradual dose tapering can be started [69]:

- dose is reduced by 10 mg every 2 weeks to 20 mg;
- thereafter, the dose is reduced by 2.5 mg every 2–4 weeks to 10 mg;
- finally it is reduced by 1 mg every 1–2 months provided there is no relapse.

Prevention of osteoporosis (calcium, vitamin D and bisphosphonate) and gastrointestinal protection (proton pump inhibitors) should be considered, since glucocorticoid therapy is generally prolonged for several years (5–6 on average) [70]. In order to reduce steroid-related untoward effects, adjunct of other immunosuppressors has been tested. Only one published trial used azathioprine to this purpose, with the result of reducing the total dose of steroids administered over 52 weeks, however with a high rate of withdrawal because of azathioprine side-effects [71]. Methotrexate adjunctive therapy was tested in GCA patients three studies with conflicting results [72–74]: however, a meta-analysis including those three studies revealed that methotrexate allowed a significant reduction in the cumulative dose of corticosteroids at 48 weeks of therapy, but not in the frequency of adverse events, and significantly

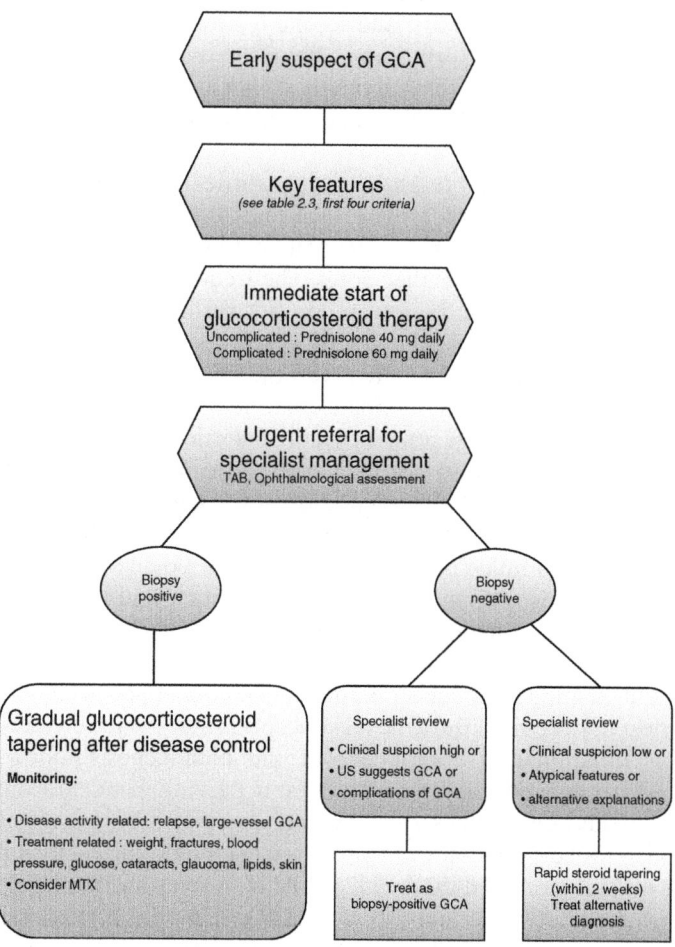

FIGURE 2.4 Schematic flowchart of diagnosis and treatment initiation for giant cell arteritis. Note that the existence of forms with negative temporal artery biopsy prompts to commence treatment even before a specialist review has confirmed the diagnosis (Modified and readapted from Ref. [69] by permission of Oxford University Press on behalf of the British Society of Rheumatology)

reduced the risk of a first and second relapse [75]. In those trials, of note, methotrexate was administered at doses between 7.5 and 15 mg/week, throughout the follow-up period (mean 55 weeks), whereas it has been suggested that higher doses (20–25 mg/week) should be evaluated in GCA patients [75].

GCA patients presenting with aortic involvement are treated with corticosteroids at the same doses as patients with cranial GCA, although it is currently not known whether they would benefit from higher doses. The frequent occurrence of aortic aneurysm, and, more rarely but earlier in the natural history, of aortic dissection in GCA patients suggests that corticosteroid doses sufficient to revert the signs and symptoms of temporal arteritis may be inadequate to suppress or prevent vasculitis of the large arteries. Data on aortic complications in patients under steroid treatment are sparse and based on small series, however the emergence of novel adjuvant therapies (including TNF-α-antagonists and IL-6 receptor antibodies; *see next section*) holds promise to address the possible need for more effective suppression of the immunitary and inflammatory response in large-vessel forms of GCA. Indeed, the improvement in the knowledge of GCA pathophysiology has brought about new concepts affecting treatment protocols. The most important of those novel concepts is that the local vascular inflammatory component of the pathogenesis follows mechanisms of development at least in part independent from those underlying the systemic immune response. Vasculitis has been found to persist even after systemic syndrome remission with glucocorticoid therapy [76], and IL-6 levels increase after discontinuation of steroids, suggesting that the usual doses given to patients induce a rapid remission of the systemic inflammatory response, even though the local arteritis persists for a greater duration [77].

Aspirin has been suggested in addition to steroid therapy, with the aim to reduce ischemic complications, however with contrasting evidences from non-randomized studies [78, 79]. Experimentally, aspirin has been shown to suppress IFN-γ transcription and enhance the suppression exerted by dexamethasone in GCA lesions [80], therefore it has been suggested to also have a possible immuno-modulating effect; whether it can be useful within steroid-sparing strategies needs to be confirmed in clinical controlled trials. A low dose (75–150 mg/day) is today recommended by the EULAR [53] in all GCA patients unless contraindications exist.

Since there is no completed placebo-controlled randomized clinical trial, the level of evidence for the management of *Takayasu's Arteritis* is low, generally reflecting the results of open studies, case series and expert opinion [53, 81–83]. The first-line medical treatment of TKA includes corticosteroids and conventional immunosuppressive agents, such as methotrexate, mycophenolate mofetil (MMF), azathioprine, cyclophosphamide. In patients who remain resistant and/or intolerant to these therapies, biologic agents (*see next section*) appear a promising adjunct. Antiplatelet treatment may lower the frequency of ischemic events in patients with TA [81–83].

The EULAR recommendation of starting therapy with 1 mg/kg/day of prednisolone or equivalent applies also to TKA treatment. As for GCA, such treatment must commence as soon as the diagnosis is done. The initial dose is maintained for at least 1 month, then if symptoms of active disease show resolve and acute-phase reactants normalize, doses are gradually tapered. A suggested tapering protocol includes [82]:

- reduction by 5 mg/week to reach 20 mg/day;
- reduction by 2.5 mg/week to reach 10 mg/day;
- reduction by 1 mg/week until discontinuation.

During steroid tapering it is quite common to observe relapses of the inflammatory activity: these are usually managed by up-titration of steroids and/or adjunction of immunosuppression. There is no evidence showing which of the different immunosuppressive agents is superior in the treatment of TKA, as no randomized study has compared their efficacy. Since methotrexate is inexpensive, easily available and relatively safe, it represents the first choice of many physicians (0.3 mg/kg/week, up to 15 mg/week) [84]. Methotrexate should be accompanied with folic acid 1 mg/day and trimethoprim/sulfamethoxazole double strength three times per week for prophylaxis against *Pneumocystis* pneumonia. Azathioprine is usually commenced at a dose of 2 mg/kg/day, MMF at 1.5 g twice per day and cyclophosphamide at 2 mg/kg/day [53, 82]. When the adjunct of immunosuppression fails to maintain disease remission, then TKA is classically considered to be refractory to conventional therapy. More recently, a Turkish study [85] defined refractory disease as angiographic or clinical progression despite treatment or the presence of any of the following characteristics: (1) prednisolone dose >7.5 mg/day after 6 months of treatment, despite administration of conventional immunosuppressive agents; (2) new surgery due to persistent disease activity; (3) frequent attacks (more than three per year) and (4) death associated with disease activity.

Of note, the rate of need for surgical revascularization in patients with stenotic evolution of arterial vasculitis can be high (about 70 %) notwithstanding good response to therapy in terms of inflammatory activity, which is achieved in as high as 60–80 % patients, regardless of the duration of remission; however, about 50 % of patients who present a first remission, can experience at least one relapse episode [81–83]. Novel vascular lesions are also observed in patients who received timely diagnosis and underwent prompt treatment, and the common belief of experts is that currently established medical treatments for TKA are severely flawed. In this perspective, the relatively low rate of disease relapse that have been reported in patients receiving adjuvant biologic agents, such as anti-TNF-α therapy, is noteworthy (*see next section*) [86]. However, confirmation of these observations in rigorous randomized controlled studies is warranted.

As for aortitis associated with GCA and TKA, also aortitis associated with other vasculitides and systemic rheumatic syndromes is treated by the same pharmacologic protocols as the primary disease. Even for those conditions that more frequently present with aortic involvement (e.g. ankylosing spondylitis, Cogan's syndrome, Behçet's disease), no specific treatment modifications are contemplated when the aorta is involved. Pharmacotherapy is based on glucocorticoids and immunosuppressive agents, whereas biologic agents are being tested in either experimental or already clinical settings, but they do not have a well-established role yet. The use of initial high dose intra-venous corticosteroids (methylprednisolone, 15 mg/kg of ideal body weight/day for the first 3 days) has been found in a single small randomized controlled trial [87] to allow for more rapid tapering of oral steroids and higher frequency of patients experiencing sustained remission of their disease after discontinuation of treatment, in the setting of GCA. This protocol is today incorporated in the official recommendations [53, 69] for complicated GCA, but independent of aortic involvement: whether it could be advantageous in this specific severe form and in the other non-infectious forms of aortitis is still to be investigated.

Novel Therapies for Non-infectious Aortitis

Glucocorticoids are the keystone of medical treatment for aortitis, but this disease is still affected by a high incidence of morbidity, and even mortality, because of the disease and its treatment. During the initial treatment with high dose glucocorticoids a dramatic improvement of symptoms is usually observed, but still a high incidence of side effects is ascribed to steroid agents, such as bone fractures, avascular necrosis of the hip, diabetes mellitus, infections, hypertension, gastro-intestinal hemorrhage, posterior sub-capsular cataract and hypertension [70]. Not of secondary importance, long term steroid therapy may affect connective tissue remodeling inside the aortic media, thus being a concomitant cause of aneurysm development and dissection occurrence in the setting of rheumatic aortitis [88]. For this reasons, the need for novel therapeutic strategies has been advocated, in order to safely allow steroids tapering and minimize the risk of disease relapse.

The last frontier is represented by biologic agents, that are immunoglobulins targeted against inflammatory mediators such as TNF-α, IL-6, IL-1, IFN-γ, or their receptors (Fig. 2.5): for some of them, the data available on their chronic use in vasculitides potentially involving the aorta are absolutely

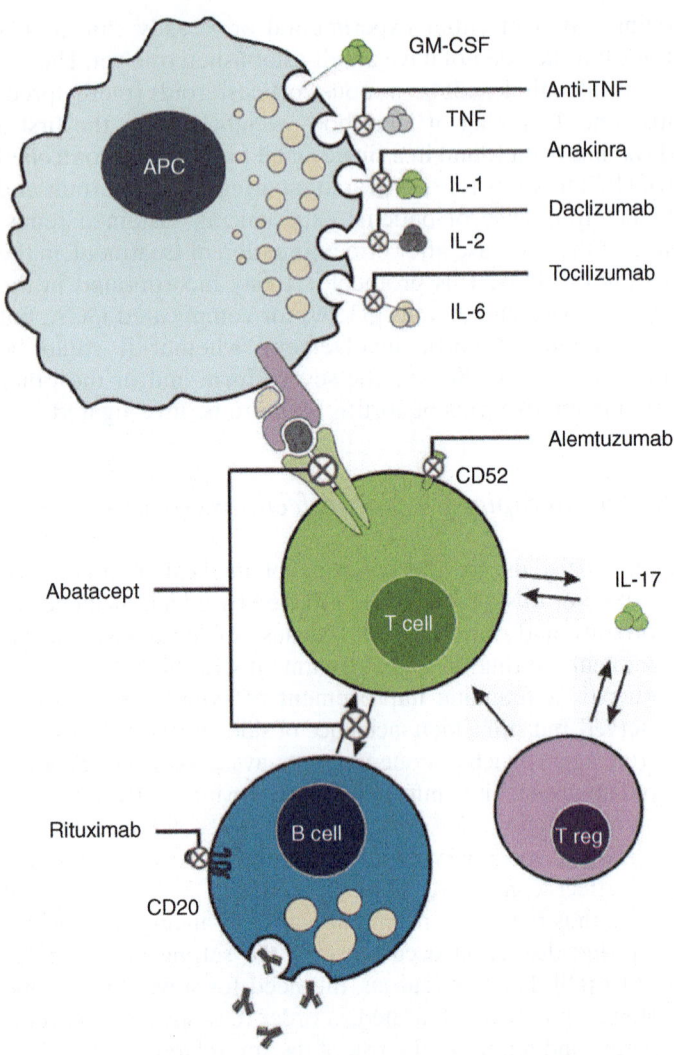

FIGURE 2.5 Cartoon depiction of the immune response steps targeted by different classes of biologic agents. Of those here represented, anti-TNF-α agents and the immunomodulator rituximab have been both employed as adjuvant therapies in large-vessel vasculitides (From Amezcua-Guerra [89])

preliminary and, although promising, the results still need confirmation in large series.

Anti-TNF-α molecules have been experimented in GCA and TKA, after the evidence of a pathogenic role for TNF-α in granulomatous inflammation. TNF-α is a product of different white blood cells involved in the chronic inflammation such as macrophages, T-cells, and natural killer (NK) cells. With an autocrine mechanism, TNF-α stimulates macrophages to produce IL-12 and IL-18 that contribute to amplify the inflammatory response acting on CD4+ T-lymphocyte differentiation and NK cells activation. IFN-γ production that leads to macrophages recruitment and activation on the inflammation site, is itself stimulated by IL-18 [86]. High circulating levels of TNF-α have been reported in GCA and TKA, and TNF-α is expressed by macrophages and dendritic cells in granulomatous vascular infiltrates, suggesting that this cytokine might be responsible for both systemic and local manifestations of the disease [90, 91] and providing the rational for anti-TNF-α therapy in both GCA and TKA.

There are three commercially available anti-TNF-α agents: *etanercept, infliximab* and *adalimumab*. Etanercept is a fusion protein of two subunits of the TNF receptor with the Fc portion of human IgG1. Infliximab is a murine-human chimeric monoclonal IgG1 antibody that binds to human TNF, causing its inactivation. Adalimumab is a recombinant, fully human IgG1 monoclonal anti-TNF-α antibody that specifically binds to the cytokine, blocking its interaction with the cell surface TNF receptors and thereby modulating TNF-induced or -modulated biological responses. The majority of the studies about the use of anti-TNF-α in large-vessel vasculitides assessed the effects of etanercept or infliximab; currently, there are limited data on the use of adalimumab to treat any form of vasculitis [92, 93]. A randomized, placebo-controlled, double-blind, multicenter trial was published, aiming at determining whether in patient with newly diagnosed GCA infliximab (5 mg/kg at weeks 0 and 6, and every 8 weeks thereafter), added to a standardized glucocorticoid protocol therapy, would provide benefits in terms of relapses, steroid doses and toxicity. The study was prematurely stopped because an interim analysis showed no significant effect of infliximab on any of the outcome variables of the study, while there was a non-significant trend for more infections in the infliximab than in the placebo group [92]. TNF-α inhibitors have proved more effective in patients with longstanding, relapsing GCA. Seventeen patients affected by biopsy-proven GCA, controlled by conventional therapy but presenting steroid-related comorbidities, were randomized to receive etanercept (25 mg twice a week subcutaneously) or placebo, and therefore glucocorticoids were tapered following a fixed schedule. Efficacy analysis showed that 50 % of the patients in the etanercept group compared to 22 % in the placebo group reached the primary end point of glucocorticoid withdrawal at 12 months. Etanercept group also had a significant lower dose of accumulated prednisone and a minor percentage of patients in this group suffered from relapses. These differences, however, did not reach statistical significance, possibly owing to the small sample size. These results suggest that etanercept may be beneficial and well tolerated in the subgroup of GCA patients with GC-refractory disease [93].

A promising preliminary evidence of TNF modulators efficacy in Takayasu's arteritis has been observed in two open-label small studies [86, 94]. Sixty-seven percent of 15 patients with steroid-resistant TKA treated with anti-TNF-α therapies achieved sustained remission of disease that lasted 1–3.3 years [86]. The long-term efficacy and safety of anti-TNF-α therapy was thereafter assessed in 25 patients with refractory TKA treated with either etanercept (25–50 mg twice a week) or infliximab (at initial dose of 3–5 mg/kg every 8 weeks): remission was achieved and prednisone was discontinued in 60 % of patients and successfully tapered below 10 mg/day in an additional 28 % of patients, while 9 out of 18 patients treated with other immunosuppressive agents could taper or discontinue the additional agent [94]. Verifying the efficacy of anti-TNF therapy in a larger randomized trial will be crucially important.

Another molecule involved in the transition from acute to chronic inflammation is IL-6. This cytokine triggers the synthesis of acute phase proteins, promotes the activation, proliferation and differentiation of different lines of T-cell lymphocytes and also leads the terminal differentiation of B cells, prolongs the survival of plasma-cells and stimulates monocytes, endothelial and stromal cells to take part in the inflammatory process [95]. Both in GCA and in TKA, IL-6 levels, both circulating and in the vessel, correlate with the activity phase of the disease. Based on this evidence, the humanized monoclonal IL-6 receptor antagonist *tocilizumab* has been proposed as a new treatment for large-vessel vasculitis, to limit auto-reactive lymphocyte differentiation in the affected vessels.

There are in the literature only case reports and very small series of tocilizumab treatment in patients affected by GCA (mostly refractory forms, but also few newly diagnosed disease cases), for a total of about 20 patients. Most common tocilizumab dosage used in those studies was 8 mg/kg every 4 weeks. The agent proved to be effective in lowering steroid dosage and in obtaining a 2-to-6-month relapse-free interval after tocilizumab discontinuation. Tocilizumab has been tolerated without major adverse events, and common side effects were cytopenia and increased levels of liver enzymes. However, persisting histological inflammation has been reported, suggesting that although tocilizumab may lead to symptomatic improvement, it is not curative [96].

In patients affected by TKA, IL-6 might be involved both in the early stage of the disease, stimulating T-cell differentiation and recruiting monocytes, and at the later stage in the processes of angiogenesis and fibrosis. There are 17 fully published cases of tocilizumab therapy in TA mostly refractory to high doses of GC and other concomitant immunosuppressive therapies. The introduction of tocilizumab achieved disease control in all patients, and helped to reduce GC dosage after 3–6 months of combined therapy. Only three cases of relapses occurred while still on tocilizumab, another one relapsed after 3 months of discontinuation of the therapy [97].

Regarding monitoring of disease activity during therapy with tocilizumab, it should be noted that anti IL-6R molecules act directly on the liver, to block the production of acute phase proteins. Therefore, monitoring should rely on clinical and radiological findings more than on the currently available laboratory markers.

B-lymphocytes represent an attractive target for providing more specific immunosuppression in the setting of vasculitis. In animal models, B-cells have been shown to be necessary not only for the development of diseases traditionally thought to be antibody driven, but also for diseases in which B-cells were believed to play a minor role. B-cells are not only the precursors of plasmacells, but they also exert "antibody-independent" functions influencing the immune response [98], including the expression of co-stimulatory molecules and release of mediators that drive CD4+ response, T-reg differentiation and maintenance of T-cell memory. Presence of B-cells has been demonstrated in affected vessels of GCA patients, thus they might be pathogenetic [7]. Also in TKA, a role for B lymphocytes has been postulated, based on the evidence of inflammatory infiltrates from aortic specimens containing B-cells and of anti-endothelium antibodies levels in the serum reflecting disease activity; moreover, an increased number of circulating plasmablasts and memory B cells have been reported in the active phase of the disease [96].

Rituximab is a chimeric IgG1 antibody that binds to CD20 expressed on the surface of B-lymphocytes and depletes circulating naive and memory B cells for 6–12 months via FcgR-mediated antibody dependent cell cytotoxicity and complement dependent cytotoxicity.

One single patient report is available demonstrating dramatic response to rituximab (1,000 mg) preceded by methylprednisolone intravenously (100 mg) in a patient previously showing relapsing GCA on high dosage of prednisone plus intravenous cyclophosphamide (500 mg). A drop in the B lymphocyte count was observed, associated with symptom improvement and disease remission confirmed both by laboratory markers and 18FDG-PET imaging, maintained for the entire follow-up time of 6 months [99].

The use of rituximab in TKA is reported in three case series with good results in five of six patients, all refractory to previous therapy with multiple immunosuppressive agents. Although promising, the very limited number of patients and the short follow-up (the longest one being 14 months) calls for further investigations to better understand the real impact of rituximab in this setting [96].

In the recently expanding pharmacological armamentarium against large-vessel vasculitis, also *leflunomide* has been introduced, an immunomodulating agent already widely used in rheumatoid arthritis, that interferes with dendritic cell maturation, reducing the production of pro-inflammatory cytokines and T-cells stimulation. Leflunomide can reduce IL-6 levels, known to be elevated in large vessel vasculitis, but unlike tocilizumab, it is orally administered and less expensive.

In a case series, leflunomide at doses of 10–20 mg was used as adjunctive therapy on 23 patients with difficult-to-treat GCA and *polymyalgia reumatica*. It was well tolerated, with favorable impact on both clinical and laboratory picture and helped steroid tapering in the majority of cases [100]. In a recent prospective study leflunomide was used at 20 mg/day in 15 patients with TA whose disease was refractory to GC and other immunosuppressant agents. Twelve patients had a favorable clinical response, i.e. a reduction of disease activity scores, CPR levels and dose of prednisone after a mean treatment duration of 9 months. However, two patients had imaging evidence of relapses, and at the end of follow-up the mean daily prednisone dose in the entire series was still superior to 10 mg [101].

Concerning the other, rarer forms of vasculitis that can be accompanied by aortitis, also in Cogan's syndrome (*see One definition for multiple diseases: classification, epidemiology, etiopathogenesis of this chapter*) novel biological therapies have been used: etanercept proved not effective in preserving hearing loss, however, it improved word identification and recognition; infliximab appeared to be effective in inducing and maintaining remission in patients with therapy-resistant CS, and it is believed to provide even greater benefit when initiated at an early stage of the disease [14]. The successful use of infliximab, adalimumab and also rituximab in single case reports of patients with relapsing-polychondritis-associated aortitis (*see first section*) has been reported, however not always capable to prevent aortic aneurysm development [102]. A metaanalysis including 20 studies with data from 3,096 patients affected by ankylosing spondylitis confirmed the beneficial effect of adjunctive therapy with TNF-α blockers in terms of both disease activity and functional capacity [103]. A promising opportunity for the use of anti-TNF-α therapy in Behçet-disease-associated vasculitides (*see first section*) arises from a number of studies that mainly evaluated this therapy in the setting of ocular inflammation. However, until results from adequately powered, randomized trials become available, anti-TNF-α agents should continue to be used with caution in BD, and their use should be limited to those patients with severe manifestations that have not responded to traditional treatments [102, 104].

Further studies are needed for a comprehensive knowledge of the immunopathogenetic mechanism of the individual vasculitides possibly involving the aorta, in order to identify new biomarkers to monitor disease activity and find new potential targets for pharmacotherapy. Studies are also warranted to establish with a higher level of evidence the role of biological agents in the adjuvant treatment of the large-vessel forms of vasculitides.

Pharmacotherapy in Infectious Aortitis

Antibiotic therapy is a fundamental part of the treatment of infectious aortitis, along with surgery. As soon as diagnosis is suspected, intravenous antibiotics should be initiated with broad antimicrobial coverage, even before microbiologic results are available. Later, antibiotic therapy may be shift accordingly to the microorganisms identified form blood cultures and their antibiotic susceptibility. If there is no high risk of impending aortic rupture, it is reasonable to start antibiotics for 2–4 weeks before surgery to improve local infection and therefore reducing the risk of post-operative infective complications [105].

There is no consensus concerning length of antibiotic therapy because it depends on surgical treatment, bacteria, aortic localization, and patient's risk factors. Commonly antibiotics are prolonged for 6–12 weeks after surgical debridement, or even longer in case of immunosuppressed patients, or persistent positive blood cultures and high biochemical parameters of inflammation. Some authors recommend life-long antibiotics in cases of difficult microorganisms or in situ prosthetic bypass [105]. Despite aggressive therapy, mortality associated with infectious aortitis remains high, mostly due to a high rate of aortic rupture.

Non-typhoid Salmonella spp., reported to be the most frequent causative microorganisms for infectious aortitis, are susceptible to fluoroquinolones and third generation cephalosporins. High-dose bactericidal therapy should be maintained for at least 6 weeks after the operation. Subsequently, long-term suppressive therapy with a bactericidal antibiotic should be used [106].

For systemic streptococcal infection a synergistic bactericidal association of benzylpenicillin (or vancomycin in cases of penicillin resistance) with gentamicin is usually administered [107]. Vaccination with polysaccharidic multivalent vaccine is recommended, notably for immunodeficient patients, to prevent mycotic aneurysm caused by *S. pneumoniae* [41].

For severe staphylococcal infections, flucoxacilline is the antibiotherapy of choice, in association, especially as start therapy, with gentamicin or oral fusidic acid or rifampicin. Erythromycin, vancomycin or parental cephalosporine can be considered in case of penicillin allergy [108].

Late syphilis is treated with penicillin G bezathine, 2.4 million units i.m. weekly for a total of three administrations. Doxycycline or ceftriaxone can be used as an alternative protocol in case of documented penicillin allergy [109].

Mycobacterial aortitis is rare and antibiotic treatment should follow the therapeutic scheme provided for general mycobacterial infections, with an association of isoniazid (300 mg/day three times weekly), rifampicin (450–600 mg/day three times weekly), pyrazinamide (1.5–2 g/day three times weekly) and also ethambutol (15 mg/kg weekly) in cases of suspected drug-resistant organisms, for a total of 2 months of treatment. The continuation therapy should be maintained for 4 months with isoniazid and rifampicin [110].

The Role of Invasive Treatment in Aortitis

Immunosuppressive drugs and antibiotics are the mainstay of the treatment of non-infectious and infectious aortitis respectively and no invasive treatment is required for non-complicated aortitis under medical treatment. However, when complications occur, invasive treatment is the only possible approach: such complications include chronic aneurysmal dilatation (more often of the aorta itself) and progressive stenosis (more often of its branches). Acute complications are represented by the life-threatening occurrence of acute aortic rupture or dissection, with or without aneurysm, and by stroke.

In non-infectious aortitis, the indications to invasive treatment do not differ from those for other etiologies causing similar complications, such as degenerative aneurysms or atherosclerotic stenosis. Both surgical and endovascular approaches have been applied in the management of aortic complications of aortitis, both for the prevention of aortic catastrophes and for the relief of chronic ischemic organ damage [111]. However, with both approaches, all guidelines concord in recommending elective surgery during the remission phase of the inflammatory disease: when emergency interventions are performed without previously controlling the inflammatory process, postoperative complications such as anastomotic dehiscence, pseudoaneurysm and restenosis are frequent [32, 53, 69].

In Takayasu's arteritis, it has been estimated that the need for invasive treatment is encountered in at least 50 % of patients under immunosuppressive therapy [112], in some cases even in apparent remission phase. The longer the follow-up after anti-inflammatory/immunosuppressive treatment start, the higher the rate of complications requiring surgery or endovascular therapy, reaching as high as 70 % over a mean period of 3 years [82]. There are no randomized trials of surgical versus endovascular treatment in TKA-associated aortitis.

Concerning stenotic lesions, percutaneous trans-luminal angioplasty (PTA) was widely used for relief of short-segment lesions, and initial reports revealed excellent results [113]; however, since restenosis can occur in more than three-fourths of the procedures, PTA might be better used only in selected cases [81]. It has been suggested that endovascular aortic repair (EVAR) can be advantageous inasmuch as it isolates a tract of the vessel wall from flow, by covering it with a stent graft, with a possible benefit for the inflammatory process [114]: reported restenosis rate is 17 % over 2 postoperative years [115]. Some authors also administer aspirin and clopidogrel perioperatively, to reduce the incidence of restenosis [81]. Surgical intervention has been demonstrated to improve long-term survival in TKA, with restenosis rates ranging between 8 and 30 % during 6 postoperative years [116], and it is considered the treatment of choice in the presence of long-segment stenosis, extensive periarterial fibrosis or complete occlusion. However, the results of bypass surgery in TKA are worse than in atherosclerotic occlusive disease, also due to the existence of clinically silent but locally active forms of vasculitis [117].

The presence of aneurysmal evolution, compared to stenosis, is a more unfavorable condition in TKA, with respect to surgical results: anastomotic pseudoaneurysm has been reported in up to 12 % patients only 2 years following surgery [118]: this prompts continuous and assiduous clinical and imaging surveillance of patients in the postoperative long-term.

When GCA is complicated by axillary or subclavian artery stenosis or occlusion, treatment involves surgical revascularization, with arterial bypass grafting from the common carotid artery, more often than EVAR, since stenosis in GCA usually involves longer segments. [119]. Open aortic reconstructive surgery is generally the standard of treatment also for aortic aneurysms associated with GCA, although endovascular techniques have been used [120]. Although endovascular treatment has the theoretical advantage of avoiding extensive manipulation of inflamed aortic tissue, there have been no head-to-head trials of the optimal strategy for managing aortic aneurysm in patients with aortitis.

Idiopathic aortitis, when complicated by inflammatory aneurysm of either thoracic or abdominal aorta, requires surgical operation, which in such cases usually results more technically demanding than in other forms of aortitis, owing to the hostile operative field with usual abundant peri-aneurysmal fibrosis and adherence with surrounding structures [121]. Consequently, perioperative mortality is threefold increased compared to surgery for other aortitides. EVAR has been demonstrated to be safer, although with higher rates of reoperations in the follow-up, mainly due to endoleaks [121].

An infectious aortitis is usually discovered late, compared to the time of onset of the infective process, and generally when diagnosis is made a mycotic aneurysm has already developed. Therefore, although antibiotherapy can "sterilize" an infected aneurysm, the definitive treatment, aimed at preventing potentially lethal rupture, is surgical, and surgery is usually required during the same hospitalization as for initial medical treatment [24]. The indications for mycotic aneurysm management do not differ from those for other aortic aneurysms (i.e. aortic diameter exceeding 5.5 cm) [28]. Two different approaches exist in surgery for infective aortitis, namely extra-anatomical bypass and direct repair with interposed grafts. The bypass approach, with debridement and ligation of the infected (generally abdominal) aorta, offers the advantage of being less prone to dehiscence and recurrence of infection, since the grafts are brought through uninfected tissue, however they imply a risk of graft thrombosis with consequent need for reoperation. Graft interposition, with removal of the affected segment, is the procedure of choice today, implying however a higher risk of early graft infection. This latter complication seems less likely to occur with the use of human allografts than with prosthetic grafts [122]. EVAR has been proposed and applied also in infectious aortitis and aneurysms, and a meta-analysis including

48 patients showed a 12-month mortality of 10 %, lower than with surgery. However reinfection of the treated segment, especially in *Salmonella spp.* infections, can occur and it carries a very high incremental risk of mortality, since surgical removal of the endograft is needed. Randomized trials to define the best invasive treatment approach to infective aortitis are still lacking [105].

References

1. Gornik HL, Creager MA. Aortitis. Circulation. 2008;117: 3039–51.

2. Jennette JC, Falk RJ, Bacon PA, Basu N, Cid MC, Ferrario F, et al. 2012 revised International Chapel Hill Consensus Conference nomenclature of vasculitides. Arthritis Rheum. 2013;65:1–11.

3. Slobodin G, Naschitz JE, Zuckerman E, Zisman D, Rozenbaum M, Boulman N, et al. Aortic involvement in rheumatic diseases. Clin Exp Rheumatol. 2006;24(2 Suppl 41):S41–7.

4. Salvarani C, Crowson CS, O'Fallon WM, Hunder GG, Gabriel SE. Reappraisal of the epidemiology of giant cell arteritis in Olmsted County, Minnesota, over a fifty-year period. Arthritis Rheum. 2004;51:264–8.

5. Hunder GG. Epidemiology of giant-cell arteritis. Cleve Clin J Med. 2002;69 Suppl 2:SII79–82.

6. Cid MC, Merkel PA. Giant cell arteritis. In: Creager M, Beckman J, Loscalzo J, editors. Vascular medicine: a companion to Braunwald's heart disease. 2nd ed. Saunders (USA); 2012. p. 525–32.

7. Weyand CM, Tetzlaff N, Björnsson J, Brack A, Younge B, Goronzy JJ. Disease patterns and tissue cytokine profiles in giant cell arteritis. Arthritis Rheum. 1997;40:19–26.

8. Maksimowicz-McKinnon K, Hoffman GS. Takayasu's arteritis. In: Creager M, Beckman J, Loscalzo J, editors. Vascular medicine: a companion to Braunwald's heart disease. 2nd ed. Saunders (USA); 2012. p. 520–4.

9. Langford CA: Takayasu's arteritis. In: Hochberg MC, Silman AJ, Smolen JS, Weinblatt ME, Weisman MH, editors. Rheumatology. 3rd ed. Mosby (USA); 2003.

10. Gravanis MB. Giant cell arteritis and Takayasu aortitis: morphologic, pathogenetic and etiologic factors. Int J Cardiol. 2000;75 Suppl 1:S21–33.

11. Bennett DL, Ohashi K, El-Khoury GY. Spondyloarthropathies: ankylosing spondylitis and psoriatic arthritis. Radiol Clin North Am. 2004;42:121–34.

12. Palazzi C, Salvarani C, D'Angelo S, Olivieri I. Aortitis and periaortitis in ankylosing spondylitis. Joint Bone Spine. 2011;78:451–5.

13. St Clair EW, McCallum RM. Cogan's syndrome. Curr Opin Rheumatol. 1999;11:47–52.

14. Greco A, Gallo A, Fusconi M, Magliulo G, Turchetta R, Marinelli C, et al. Cogan's syndrome: an autoimmune inner ear disease. Autoimmun Rev. 2013;12:396–400.

15. Tseng JF, Cambria RP, Aretz HT, Brewster DC. Thoracoabdominal aortic aneurysm in Cogan's syndrome. J Vasc Surg. 1999; 30:565–8.

16. Gürgün C, Ercan E, Ceyhan C, Yavuzgil O, Zoghi M, Aksu K, et al. Cardiovascular involvement in Behçet's disease. Jpn Heart J. 2002;43:389–98.

17. Hamza M. Large artery involvement in Behçet's disease. J Rheumatol. 1987;14:554–9.

18. Chae EJ, Do KH, Seo JB, Park SH, Kang JW, Jang YM, et al. Radiologic and clinical findings of Behçet disease: comprehensive review of multisystemic involvement. Radiographics. 2008;28:e31.

19. Chirinos JA, Tamariz LJ, Lopes G, Del Carpio F, Zhang X, Milikowski C, et al. Large vessel involvement in ANCA-associated vasculitides: report of a case and review of the literature. Clin Rheumatol. 2004;23:152–9.

20. Tavora F, Burke A. Review of isolated ascending aortitis: differential diagnosis, including syphilitic, Takayasu's and giant cell aortitis. Pathology. 2006;38:302–8.

21. Restrepo CS, Ocazionez D, Suri R, Vargas D. Aortitis: imaging spectrum of the infectious and inflammatory conditions of the aorta. Radiographics. 2011;31:435–51.

22. Stone JR. Aortitis, periaortitis, and retroperitoneal fibrosis, as manifestations of IgG4-related systemic disease. Curr Opin Rheumatol. 2011;23:88–94.

23. Foote EA, Postier RG, Greenfield RA, Bronze MS. Infectious aortitis. Curr Treat Options Cardiovasc Med. 2005;7:89–97.

24. Valentine RJ, Plummer MM. Vascular infections. In: Creager M, Beckman J, Loscalzo J, editors. Vascular medicine: a companion to Braunwald's heart disease. 2nd ed. Saunders (USA); 2012. 709–26.

25. Gomes MN, Choyke PL, Wallace RB. Infected aortic aneurysms: a changing entity. Ann Surg. 1992;215:435–42.

26. Schmidt WA, Gromnica-Ihle E. What is the best approach to diagnosing large-vessel vasculitis? Best Pract Res Clin Rheumatol. 2005;19:223–42.

27. Hunder GG, Bloch DA, Michel BA, Stevens MB, Arend WP, Calabrese LH, et al. The American College of Rheumatology 1990 criteria for the classification of giant cell arteritis. Arthritis Rheum. 1990;33:1122–8.

28. Bossert M, Prati C, Balblanc JC, Lohse A, Wendling D. Aortic involvement in giant cell arteritis: current data. Joint Bone Spine. 2011;78:246–51.

29. Nuenninghoff DM, Hunder GG, Christianson TJ, McClelland RL, Matteson EL. Incidence and heumattors of large-artery complication (aortic aneurysm, aortic dissection, and/or large-artery stenosis) in patients with giant cell arteritis: a population-based study over 50 years. Arthritis Rheum. 2003;48:3522–31.

30. Scheel AK, Meller J, Vosshenrich R, Kohlhoff E, Siefker U, Müller GA, et al. Diagnosis and follow up of aortitis in the elderly. Ann Rheum Dis. 2004;63:1507–10.

31. Johnston SL, Lock RJ, Gompels MM. Takayasu arteritis: a review. J Clin Pathol. 2002;55:481–6.

32. Hiratzka LF, Bakris GL, Beckman JA, Bersin RM, Carr VF, Casey Jr DE, et al. 2010 ACCF/AHA/AATS/ACR/ASA/SCA/SCAI/SIR/STS/SVM guidelines for the diagnosis and management of patients with thoracic aortic disease: a report of the American College of Cardiology Foundation/American Heart Association Task Force on Practice Guidelines, American Association for Thoracic Surgery, American College of Radiology, American Stroke Association, Society of Cardiovascular Anesthesiologists, Society for Cardiovascular Angiography and Interventions, Society of Interventional Radiology, Society of Thoracic Surgeons, and Society for Vascular Medicine. Circulation. 2010;121:e266–369.

33. Sueyoshi E, Sakamoto I, Hayashi K. Aortic aneurysms in patients with Takayasu's arteritis: CT evaluation. AJR Am J Roentgenol. 2000;175:1727–33.

34. Tavora F, Jeudy J, Gocke C, Burke A. Takayusu aortitis with acute dissection and hemopericardium. Cardiovasc Pathol. 2005;14:320–3.

35. Arend WP, Michel BA, Bloch DA, Hunder GG, Calabrese LH, Edworthy SM, et al. The American College of Rheumatology

1990 criteria for the classification of Takayasu arteritis. Arthritis Rheum. 1990;33:1129–34.

36. Roldan CA, Chavez J, Wiest PW, Qualls CR, Crawford MH. Aortic root disease and valve disease associated with ankylosing spondylitis. J Am Coll Cardiol. 1998;32:1397–404.

37. Grasland A, Pouchot J, Hachulla E, Blétry O, Papo T, Vinceneux P. Study Group for Cogan's Syndrome. Typical and atypical Cogan's syndrome: 32 cases and review of the literature. Rheumatology (Oxford). 2004;43:1007–15.

38. Selim AG, Fulford LG, Mohiaddin RH, Sheppard MN. Active aortitis in relapsing polychondritis. J Clin Pathol. 2001;54:890–2.

39. Rojo-Leyva F, Ratliff NB, Cosgrove 3rd DM, Hoffman GS. Study of 52 patients with idiopathic aortitis from a cohort of 1,204 surgical cases. Arthritis Rheum. 2000;43:901–7.

40. Revest M, Decaux O, Cazalets C, Verohye JP, Jégo P, Grosbois B. Thoracic infectious aortitis: microbiology, pathophysiology and treatment. Rev Med Interne. 2007;28:108–15.

41. Cartery C, Astudillo L, Deelchand A, Moskovitch G, Sailler L, Bossavy JP, et al. Abdominal infectious aortitis caused by Streptococcus pneumonia: a case report and literature review. Ann Vasc Surg. 2011;25:266.e9–16.

42. Roberts WC, Ko JM, Vowels TJ. Natural history of syphilitic aortitis. Am J Cardiol. 2009;104:1578–87.

43. Merkel PA. Overview of vasculitis. In: Creager M, Beckman J, Loscalzo J, editors. Vascular medicine: a companion to Braunwald's heart disease. 2nd ed. Saunders (USA); 2012. p. 507–19.

44. Schmidt WA, Kraft HE, Borkowski A, Gromnica-Ihle EJ. Colour duplex ultrasonography in large-vessel giant cell arteritis. Scand J Rheumatol. 1999;28:374–6.

45. Schmidt WA. Imaging in vasculitis. Best Pract Res Clin Rheumatol. 2013;27:107–18.

46. Hautzel H, Sander O, Heinzel A, Schneider M, Müller HW. Assessment of large-vessel involvement in giant cell arteritis with 18 F-FDG PET: introducing an ROC-analysis-based cutoff ratio. J Nucl Med. 2008;49:1107–13.

47. Schmidt WA, Blockmans D. Use of ultrasonography and positron emission tomography in the diagnosis and assessment of large-vessel vasculitis. Curr Opin Rheumatol. 2005;17:9–15.

48. Ceriani L, Oberson M, Marone C, Gallino A, Giovanella L. F-18 FDG PET-CT Imaging in the care-management of a patient with pan-aortitis and coronary involvement. Clin Nucl Med. 2007;32:562–4.

49. Choe YH, Han BK, Koh EM, Kim DK, Do YS, Lee WR. Takayasu's arteritis: assessment of disease activity with contrast-enhanced MR imaging. AJR Am J Roentgenol. 2000; 175:505–11.

50. Schmidt WA, Nerenheim A, Seipelt E, Poehls C, Gromnica-Ihle E. Diagnosis of early Takayasu arteritis by colour Doppler ultrasonography. Rheumatology. 2002;41:496–502.

51. Roldán-Valadéz E, Hernández-Martínez P, Osorio-Peralta S, Elizalde-Acosta I, Espinoza-Cruz V, Casián-Castellanos G. Imaging diagnosis of subclavian steal syndrome secondary to Takayasu arteritis affecting a left-side subclavian artery. Arch Med Res. 2003;34:433–8.

52. Song JK, Jeong YH, Kang DH, Song JM, Song H, Choo SJ, et al. Echocardiographic and clinical characteristics of aortic regurgitation because of systemic vasculitis. J Am Soc Echocardiogr. 2003;16:850–7.

53. Mukhtyar C, Guillevin L, Cid MC, Dasgupta B, de Groot K, Gross W, et al. EULAR recommendations for the management of large vessel vasculitis. Ann Rheum Dis. 2009;68:318–23.

54. Chowdhary VR, Crowson CS, Bhagra AS, Warrington KG, Vrtiska TJ. CT angiographic imaging characteristics of thoracic idiopathic aortitis. J Cardiovasc Comput Tomogr. 2013;7: 297–302.

55. Wang H, Smith RN, Spooner AE, Isselbacher EM, Cambria RP, MacGillivray TE, et al. Giant cell aortitis of the ascending aorta without signs or symptoms of systemic vasculitis is associated with elevated risk of distal aortic events. Arthritis Rheum. 2012;64:317–9.

56. Iino M, Kuribayashi S, Imakita S, Takamiya M, Matsuo H, Ookita Y, et al. Sensitivity and specificity of CT in the diagnosis of inflammatory abdominal aortic aneurysms. J Comput Assist Tomogr. 2002;26:1006–12.

57. Cronin CG, Lohan DG, Blake MA, Roche C, McCarthy P, Murphy JM. Retroperitoneal fibrosis: a review of clinical features and imaging findings. AJR Am J Roentgenol. 2008;191:423–31.

58. Malouf JF, Chandrasekaran K, Orszulak TA. Mycotic aneurysms of the thoracic aorta: a diagnostic challenge. Am J Med. 2003;115:489–96.

59. Wein M, Bartel T, Kabatnik M, Sadony V, Dirsch O, Erbel R. Rapid progression of bacterial aortitis to an ascending aortic mycotic aneurysm documented by transesophageal echocardiography. J Am Soc Echocardiogr. 2001;14:646–9.

60. Wilson SE, Van Wagenen P, Passaro Jr E. Arterial infection. Curr Probl Surg. 1978;15:1–89.
61. Macedo TA, Stanson AW, Oderich GS, Johnson CM, Panneton JM, Tie ML. Infected aortic aneurysms: imaging findings. Radiology. 2004;231:250–7.
62. Litmanovich DE, Yıldırım A, Bankier AA. Insights into imaging of aortitis. Insights Imaging. 2012;3:545–60.
63. Huang JS, Ho AS, Ahmed A, Bhalla S, Menias CO. Borne identity: CT imaging of vascular infections. Emerg Radiol. 2011;18: 335–43.
64. Katabathina VS, Restrepo CS. Infectious and noninfectious aortitis: cross-sectional imaging findings. Semin Ultrasound CT MR. 2012;33:207–21.
65. Long R, Guzman R, Greenberg H, Safneck J, Hershfield E. Tuberculous mycotic aneurysm of the aorta: review of published medical and surgical experience. Chest. 1999;115: 522–31.
66. Kimura F, Satoh H, Sakai F, Nishii N, Tohda J, Fujimura M, et al. Computed tomographic findings of syphilitic aortitis. Cardiovasc Intervent Radiol. 2004;27:179–81.
67. Bodhey NK, Gupta AK, Neelakandhan KS, Unnikrishnan M. Early sternal erosion and luetic aneurysms of thoracic aorta: report of 6 cases and analysis of cause-effect relationship. Eur J Cardiothorac Surg. 2005;28:499–501.
68. Tomey MI, Murthy VL, Beckman JA. Giant syphilitic aortic aneurysm: a case report and review of the literature. Vasc Med. 2011;16:360–4.
69. Dasgupta B, Borg FA, Hassan N, Alexander L, Barraclough K, Bourke B, et al. BSR and BHPR guidelines for the management of giant cell arteritis. Rheumatology (Oxford). 2010;49:1594–7.
70. Proven A, Gabriel SE, Orces C, O'Fallon M, Hunder GG. Glucocorticoid therapy in giant cell arteritis: duration and adverse outcomes. Arthritis Rheum. 2003;49:703–8.
71. De Silva M, Hazleman BL. Azathioprine in giant cell arteritis/polymyalgia rheumatica: a double-blind study. Ann Rheum Dis. 1986;45:136–8.
72. Hoffman GS, Cid MC, Hellmann DB, Guillevin L, Stone JH, Schousboe J, et al., for the International Network for the Study of Systemic Vasculitides (INSSYS). A multicenter, randomized, double-blind, placebo-controlled trial of adjuvant methotrexate treatment for giant cell arteritis. Arthritis Rheum. 2002;46: 1309–18.

73. Jover JA, Hernandez-Garcia C, Morado IC, Vargas E, Banares A, Fernandez-Gutierrez B. Combined treatment of giant-cell arteritis with methotrexate and prednisone: a randomized, double-blind, placebo-controlled trial. Ann Intern Med. 2001; 134:106–14.

74. Spiera RF, Mitnick HJ, Kupersmith M, Richmond M, Spiera H, Peterson MG, et al. A prospective, double-blind, randomized, placebo controlled trial of methotrexate in the treatment of giant cell arteritis (GCA). Clin Exp Rheumatol. 2001;19:495–501.

75. Mahr AD, Jover JA, Spiera RF, Hèrnandez-Garcìa C, Fernàndez-Gutiérrez B, LaValley MP, et al. Adjunctive methotrexate for treatment of giant cell arteritis: an individual patient data meta-analysis. Arthritis Rheum. 2007;56:2789–97.

76. Achkar AA, Lie JT, Hunder GG, O'Fallon WM, Gabriel SE. How does previous corticosteroid treatment affect the biopsy findings in giant cell (temporal) arteritis? Ann Intern Med. 1994;120:987–92.

77. Weyand CM, Fulbright JW, Hunder GG, Evans JM, Goronzy JJ. Treatment of giant cell arteritis: interleukin-6 as a biologic marker of disease activity. Arthritis Rheum. 2000;43:1041–8.

78. Lee MS, Smith SD, Galor A, Hoffman GS. Antiplatelet and anticoagulant therapy in patients with giant cell arteritis. Arthritis Rheum. 2006;54:3306–9.

79. Salvarani C, Della Bella C, Cimino L, Macchioni P, Formisano D, Bajocchi G, et al. Risk factors for severe cranial ischaemic events in an Italian population-based cohort of patients with giant cell arteritis. Rheumatology (Oxford). 2009;48:250–3.

80. Weyand CM, Kaiser M, Yang H, Younge B, Goronzy JJ. Therapeutic effects of acetylsalicylic acid in giant cell arteritis. Arthritis Rheum. 2002;46:457–66.

81. Keser G, Direskeneli H, Aksu K. Management of Takayasu arteritis: a systematic review. Rheumatology. 2014;53:793–801.

82. Maximowicz-McKinnon K, Clark TM, Hoffmann GS. Limitations of therapy and a guarded prognosis in an American cohort of Takayasu arteritis patients. Arthritis Rheum. 2007; 56:1000–9.

83. Wen D, Du X, Ma CS. Takayasu arteritis: diagnosis. Treatment and prognosis. Int Rev Immunol. 2012;31:462–73.

84. Hoffman GS, Leavitt RY, Kerr GS, Rottem M, Sneller MC, Fauci AS. Treatment of glucocorticoid resistant or relapsing Takayasu arteritis with methotrexate. Arthritis Rheum. 1994; 37:578–82.

85. Saruhan-Direskeneli G, Hughes T, Aksu K, Keser G, Coit P, Aydin SZ, et al. Identification of multiple genetic susceptibility loci in Takayasu arteritis. Am J Hum Genet. 2013;93:298–305.
86. Hoffman GS, Merkel PA, Brasington RD, Lenschow DJ, Liang P. Anti–tumor necrosis factor therapy in patients with difficult to treat Takayasu arteritis. Arthritis Rheum. 2004;50:2296–304.
87. Mazlumzadeh M, Hunder GG, Easley KA, Calamia KT, Matteson EL, Griffing WL, et al. Treatment of giant cell arteritis using induction therapy with high-dose glucocorticoids: a double-blind, placebo-controlled, randomized prospective clinical trial. Arthritis Rheum. 2006;54:3310–8.
88. Ohara N, Miyata T, Sato O, Oshiro H, Shigematsu H. Aortic aneurysm in patients with autoimmune diseases treated with corticosteroids. Int Angiol. 2000;19:270–5.
89. Amezcua-Guerra LM, editor. Advances in the diagnosis and treatment of vasculitis. InTech (Croatia); 2011. ISBN 978-953-307-786-4. doi:10.5772/21534.
90. Wagner AD, Wittkop U, Prahst A, Schmidt WA, Gromnica-Ihle E, Vorpahl K, et al. Dendritic cells colocalize with activated CD4-T cells in giant cell arteritis. Clin Exp Rheumatol. 2003;21:185–92.
91. Field M, Cook A, Gallagher G. Immuno-localisation of tumour necrosis factor and its receptors in temporal arteritis. Rheumatol Int. 1997;17:113–8.
92. Hoffman GS, Cid MC, Rendt-Zagar KE, Merkel PA, Weyand CM, Stone JH, et al. Infliximab for maintenance of glucocorticosteroid-induced remission of giant cell arteritis: a randomized trial. Ann Intern Med. 2007;146:621–30.
93. Martínez-Taboada VM, Rodríguez-Valverde V, Carreño L, López-Longo J, Figueroa M, Belzunegui J, et al. A double-blind placebo controlled trial of etanercept in patients with giant cell arteritis and corticosteroid side effects. Ann Rheum Dis. 2008; 67:625–30.
94. Molloy ES, Langford CA, Clark TM, Gota CE, Hoffman GS. Anti-tumour necrosis factor therapy in patients with refractory Takayasu arteritis: long-term follow-up. Ann Rheum Dis. 2008;67:1567–9.
95. Naka T, Nishimoto N, Kishimoto T. The paradigm of IL-6: from basic science to medicine. Arthritis Res. 2002;4 Suppl 3: S233–42.
96. Unizony S, Stone JH, Stone JR. New treatment strategies in large-vessel vasculitis. Curr Opin Rheumatol. 2013;25:3–9.

97. Clifford A, Hoffman GS. Recent advances in the medical management of Takayasu arteritis: an update on use of biologic therapies. Curr Opin Rheumatol. 2014;26:7–15.

98. Lund FE, Randall TD. Effector and regulatory B cells: modulators of CD4+ T-cell immunity. Nat Rev Immunol. 2010;10:236–47.

99. Bhatia A, Ell PJ, Edwards JC. Anti-CD20 monoclonal antibody (rituximab) as an adjunct in the treatment of giant cell arteritis. Ann Rheum Dis. 2005;64:1099–100.101.

100. Adizie T, Christidis D, Dharmapaliah C, Borg F, Dasgupta B. Efficacy and tolerability of leflunomide in difficult-to-treat polymyalgia rheumatica and giant cell arteritis: a case series. Int J Clin Pract. 2012;66:906–9.

101. de Souza AW, da Silva MD, Machado LS, Oliveira AC, Pinheiro FA, Sato EI. Short-term effect of leflunomide in patients with Takayasu arteritis: an observational study. Scand J Rheumatol. 2012;41:227–30.

102. Schäfer VS, Zwerina J. Biologic treatment of large-vessel vasculitides. Curr Opin Rheumatol. 2012;24:31–7.

103. Callhoff J, Sieper J, Weiß A, Zink A, Listing J. Efficacy of TNFα blockers in patients with ankylosing spondylitis and non-radiographic axial spondyloarthritis: a meta-analysis. Ann Rheum Dis. 2014. doi:10.1136/annrheumdis-2014-205322.

104. Langford CA. Drug insight: anti-tumor necrosis factor therapies for the vasculitic diseases. Nat Clin Pract Rheumatol. 2008;4:364–70.

105. Lopes RJ, Almeida J, Dias PJ, Pinho P, Maciel MJ. Infectious thoracic aortitis: a literature review. Clin Cardiol. 2009;32:488–90.

106. Soravia-Dunand VA, Loo VG, Salit IE. Aortitis due to Salmonella: report of 10 cases and comprehensive review of the literature. Clin Infect Dis. 1999;29:862–8.

107. Wilks D, Farrington M, Rubenstein D. Streptococci and their relatives. In: The infectious diseases manual. 2nd ed. Oxford: Blackwell Science Ltd; 2008.

108. Wilks D, Farrington M, Rubenstein D. Staphylococci. In: The infectious diseases manual. 2nd ed. Oxford: Blackwell Science Ltd; 2008.

109. Cohen SE, Klausner JD, Engelman J, Philip S. Syphilis in the modern era: an update for physicians. Infect Dis Clin North Am. 2013;27:705–22.

110. Wilks D, Farrington M, Rubenstein D. Mycobacteria and mycobacterial infections. In: The infectious diseases manual. 2nd ed. Oxford: Blackwell Science Ltd; 2008.

111. Gornik HL, Creager MA. Diseases of the aorta. In: Topol EJ, editor. Textbook of cardiovascular medicine. 3rd ed. Philadelphia: Lippincott, Williams & Wilkins; 2007.

112. Vanoli M, Daina E, Salvarani C, Sabbadini MG, Rossi C, Bacchiani G, et al. Takayasu's arteritis: a study of 104 Italian patients. Arthritis Rheum. 2005;53:100–7.

113. Lee BB, Laredo J, Neville R, et al. Endovascular management of Takayasu arteritis: is it a durable option? Vascular. 2009;17:138–46.

114. Qureshi MA, Martin Z, Greenberg RK. Endovascular management of patients with Takayasu arteritis: stents versus stent Grafts. Semin Vasc Surg. 2011;24:44–52.

115. Min PK, Park S, Jung JH, et al. Endovascular therapy combined with immunosuppressive treatment for occlusive arterial disease in patients with Takayasu's arteritis. J Endovasc Ther. 2005; 12:28–34.

116. Isobe M. Takayasu arteritis revisited: current diagnosis and treatment. Int J Cardiol. 2013;168:3–10.

117. Tyagi S, Verma PK, Gambhir DS, et al. Early and long-term results of subclavian angioplasty in aortoarteritis (Takayasu disease): comparison with atherosclerosis. Cardiovasc Intervent Radiol. 1998;21:219–24.

118. Miyata T, Sato O, Deguchi J, et al. Anastomotic aneurysms after surgical treatment of Takayasu's arteritis: a 40-year experience. J Vasc Surg. 1998;27:438–45.

119. Both M, Aries PM, Muller-Hulsbeck S, Jahnke T, Schafer PJ, Gross WL, et al. Balloon angioplasty of arteries of the upper extremities in patients with extracranial giant-cell arteritis. Ann Rheum Dis. 2006;65:1124–30.

120. Baril DT, Carroccio A, Palchik E, Ellozy SH, Jacobs TS, Teodorescu V, et al. Endovascular treatment of complicated aortic aneurysms in patients with underlying arteriopathies. Ann Vasc Surg. 2006;20:464–71.

121. Puchner S, Bucek RA, Rand T, Schoder M, Hölzenbein T, Kretschmer G, Reiter M, et al. Endovascular therapy of inflammatory aortic aneurysms: a meta-analysis. J Endovasc Ther. 2005;12:560–7.

122. Brown KE, Heyer K, Rodriguez H, et al. Arterial reconstruction with cryopreserved human allografts in the setting of infection: a single-center experience with midterm follow-up. J Vasc Surg. 2009;49:660.

Chapter 3
Pharmacotherapy of Thoracic Aortic Aneurysm

Guillaume Jondeau, Olivier Milleron, Claire Bouleti, and Jean-Baptiste Michel

Aortic aneurysm is defined as a permanent focal aorta dilatation. with at least a 50 % increase in diameter compared with the expected normal diameter Thoracic aortic aneurysms (TAA) may involve one or more aortic segments (aortic root, ascending aorta, arch or descending aorta). Sixty percent of TAAs involve the aortic root and/or ascending tubular aorta, 40 % the descending aorta, 10 % the arch, and 10 % the thoracoabdominal aorta. In the ascending aorta, genetic factors are of major importance and in the descending aorta, the risk factors for atherosclerosis are of major importance.

G. Jondeau (✉)
Centre National Maladies Rares Syndrome de Marfan et apparentés, INSERM U1148 (LVTS), Université Paris 7, AP-HP Hopital Bichat, Paris 75018, France
e-mail: guillaume.jondeau@bch.aphp.fr

O. Milleron • C. Bouleti
Centre National Maladies Rares Syndrome de Marfan et apparentés, INSERM U1148 (LVTS), AP-HP Hopital Bichat, Paris 75018, France

J.-B. Michel
Centre National Maladies Rares Syndrome de Marfan et apparentés, INSERM U1148 (LVTS), Hopital Bichat, Paris 75018, France

A. Evangelista, C.A. Nienaber (eds.), *Pharmacotherapy in Aortic Disease*, Current Cardiovascular Therapy, Vol. 7, DOI 10.1007/978-3-319-09555-4_3,
© Springer International Publishing Switzerland 2015

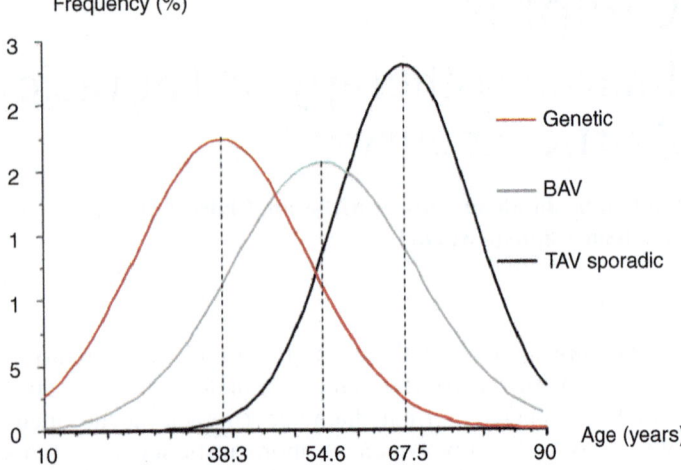

FIGURE 3.1 Age at surgery according to the type of TAA

Thoracic aortic aneurysm has an estimated incidence of approximately 10 per 100,000 person-years [1]. The natural history and treatment strategy depend on the location of the aneurysm and its underlying cause (Fig. 3.1).

Actually, available literature about TAA is limited, and there has been very few medical studies in this group of patients for several reasons:

TAA is a rare disease.

TAA is usually not responsible for any symptoms before a complication occurs.

Discovery of TAA requires imaging of the aorta, usually indicated for other reasons.

The disease is usually discovered when the dilatation is large and therefore the period of time during which a therapy can be tested is limited.

Familial screening of TAA related for genetic defects should permit early discovery of some aortic diseases. However, recognition of the genetic nature of TAA and awareness of the cardiologic community are only recent.

In the absence of a large population of patients with long follow-up, it is difficult to test a medical therapy according to medical standards (i.e. evidence based medicine). The only studies available were conducted in selected populations with TAA of genetic aetiology, such as Marfan syndrome. This approach allows for early recognition of patients "at risk" of developing TAA (since they have a genetic defect), but Marfan syndrome remains a rare disease, and the studies performed therefore included limited number of patients (cf Marfan syndrome Chap. 4 for complete discussion). To date, no medical therapy has been clearly demonstrated to be associated with decreased mortality or complication rate.

Although aneurysms reaching a certain size are generally treated with surgery or endovascular therapy, many aspects of their medical management should be considered first.

Therefore, when caring for TAA patients medically, we lack evidenced based medicine, and are left with only reasoning, as was medicine in the preceding century, i.e., an art! As a result, the proposals made below cannot be considered as established truth, and the aim of this review is discuss the current state of the art.

If reasoning is the forefront on medical therapy in a patient with TAA, the first aim should be to assess the natural history of the disease and to seek for a modifiable etiologic factor, and treat it accordingly.

In fact TAA can be due to multiple etiologies, with varying prognosis (Fig. 3.1).

Aetiologies of TAA

From family studies, it is estimated that 20 % of TAAs are due to genetic diseases. The common pattern of inheritance seems to be autosomal dominant with different penetrance levels [2]. Among other risk factors, more important for the descending thoracic aorta, smoking has the strongest association with TAA. Dyslipidemia and hypertension are less powerful risk factors, considered to be associated mainly with the occurrence of AAA, although some data suggest that hypertension may actually be more closely associated with and is certainly a risk factor for dissection [3]. Men are more often affected than women (this is true whether an aneurysm is secondary to genetic factors or not). Advanced age, hypertension, chronic obstructive lung disease, and coronary artery disease are also associated risk factors for descending TAA [4].

Genetic Forms of TAA (Predominant in the Ascending Aorta)

The most common genetic aetiology for TAA is a mutation in the *FBN1* gene, by far the most frequent cause of Marfan syndrome. Beyond *FBN1* gene mutations, other genes have been implicated in the development of TAA, and can be grouped into different categories (Montalcino Aortic Consortium Classification) [5] (Table 3.1, Fig. 3.2).

1. Mutation within genes coding for an extra-cellular matrix protein (*FBN1*, *COL3A1*). Such mutations are responsible for syndromic TAA, i.e. TAA associated with extra-aortic features (Marfan Syndrome, and vascular Ehlers Danlos syndrome).

   (a) Marfan syndrome is usually secondary to mutations in the *FBN1* gene and leads to multisystem findings including skeletal features (tall stature, scoliosis, pectus deformities, elongated fingers and toes, hyperflexibility), ocular involvement (lens dislocation, high myopia), striae atrophiae, pneumothorax, and cardiovascular disease (aortic root aneurysm, aortic dissection, mitral valve prolapse) [6, 7]. See Marfan syndrome Chap. 4

   (b) Vascular Ehlers Danlos syndrome (vEDS) can be suspected on a variety of symptoms (medium sized arterial rupture, digestive complication such as bowel perforation, uterine rupture during pregnancy [8], and is confirmed nowadays by genetic testing (presence of a mutation at the *COL3A1* gene encoding the pro-alpha 1 chain of type III procollagen. Actually, aortic

TABLE 3.1 Genetic etiologies of TAA (Montalcino Aortic Consortium)

Gene	Molecule	Phenotype
ECM		
FBN1	Fibrillin-1	Marfan syndrome
COL3A1	Type3 procollagen	Vascular Ehlers–Danlos syndrome
COL4A5	Type4 procollagen	Alport syndrome
EFEMP2	Fibulin-4	Cutis laxa
TGFβ path		
TGFBR1	TGF-β receptor-1	FTAAD/LDS
TGFBR2	TGF-β receptor-2	FTAAD/MFS/LDS
TGFB2	TGF-β2	FTAAD
SMAD3	SMAD3	FTAAD/AOS
Contractile		
ACTA2	α-actin	FTAAD
MYH11	Myosin heavy chain-11	FTAAD
MYLK	Myosin light chain kinase	FTAAD
PRKG1	cGMP-dependent	FTAAD
FLNA	Filamin-A	Cerebral heterotopias/Aortic aneurysm
TSC2	Tuberin	Tuberous sclerosis complex
Others		
JAG1	JAGGED-1	Alagille syndrome
NOTCH1	NOTCH-1	Bicuspid aortic valve/Ao aneurysm
SLC2A10	Glucose transporter 10	Arterial tortuosity syndrome

Mutations responsible for Thoracic Aortic Aneurysms are classified according to the function of the gene affected

ECM extracellular matrix, *TGFβ path* components of the TGFB pathway, *Contractile* contractile apparatus of the smooth muscle cell, *FTAAD* familial Thoracic Aortic Dissection, *LDS* Loeys Dietz syndrome, *MFS* Marfan syndrome, *AOS* aneurysm osteoarthritis syndrome

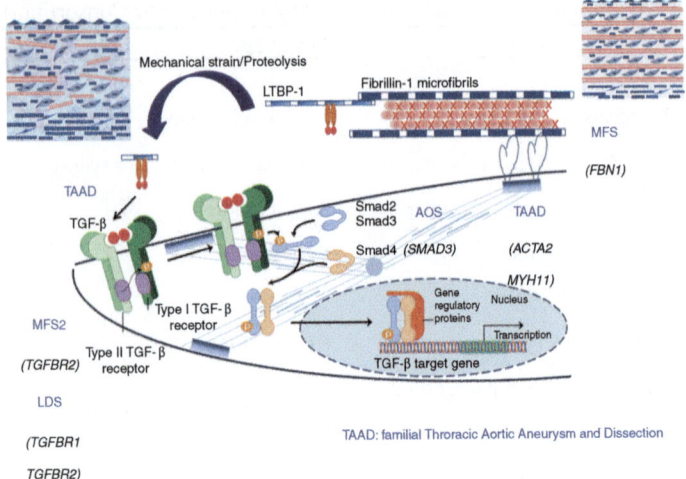

FIGURE 3.2 More frequent genetic etiologies for *TAAD* (Thoracic Aortic Aneurysm Dissection); see text for abbreviations

aneurysms are not frequent in this pathology which is more responsible for aortic dissection than dilatation.

2. Mutations within genes coding for a protein involved in the TGFB pathway (*TGFB2, TGFBR1, TGFBR2, SMAD3*), are associated with TAA but also aneurysms of other arteries, and possibly extra-aortic features (Aneurysm Osteoarthiritis Syndrome associated with *SMAD3* mutation, LDS associated with mutation in *TGFBR1* or *TGFBR2*, Marfan syndrome type II owing to *TGFBR2* mutation) (Fig. 3.3).

(a) Loeys-Dietz syndrome is a severe syndrome due to mutations in *TGFBR1* and *TGFBR2* genes and has a characteristic triad of craniofacial features (craniosynostosis, bifid uvula, hypertelorism), aortic root and branch vessel aneurysm and dissection, and arterial tortuosity [9, 10]. Mutations in *TGFBR2* can also be responsible for familial forms of TAA with dominant autosomic inheritance pattern, and incomplete penetrance [11]. They can also be responsible for skeletal features similar to that observed in MFS syndrome related to *FBN1* mutation [12].

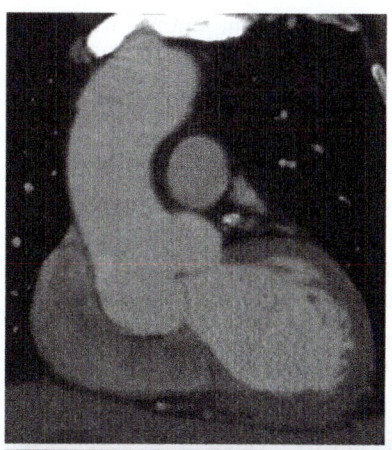

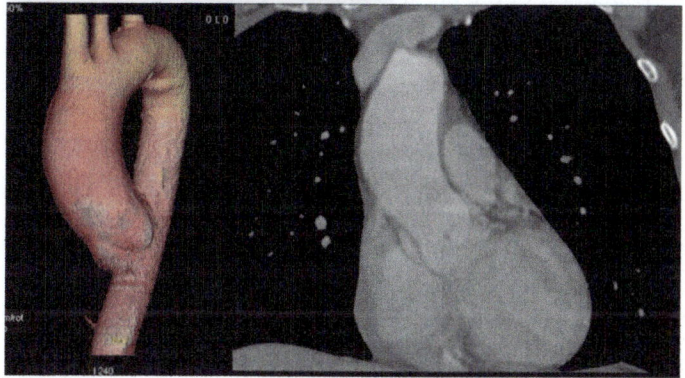

FIGURE 3.3 *Top*: aortic root dilatation in a patient with TGFB2 mutation: CT scanner. Maximal diameter at the level of the sinuses of Valsalva is 50 mm, and was considered as an indication for surgery. *Bottom*: aortic dilatation observed in a patient with a brother with BAV and TAA. Although the patient presented here did not show BAV, aortic dilatation of the tubular junction was shown on the CT scanner

   (b) Aneurysm Osteoarthritis Syndrome associates early-onset Osteoarthritis, Charcot-Marie-Tooth like neuropathy, autoimmune features, multiple arterial aneurysms and dissections [13] and secondary to *SMAD3* mutations.

   (c) *TGFB2* mutations are responsible for familial TAA with some skeletal features of Marfan Syndrome [14]

3. Mutations within genes coding for components of the contractility apparatus of the smooth muscle cell (ACTA2, MYH11, PRKG1, FLNA).

(a) *ACTA2* gene mutations affect approximately 14 % of individuals with familial TAA disease in an serie from the USA but is much less frequent in our population. These mutations can be associated with livedo reticularis, iris flocculi, cerebral aneurysms, premature coronary and cerebrovascular disease, moyamoya [15, 16].

(b) *MYH11* gene mutations are responsible for familial forms of TAA often with patent ductus arteriosus [17]. They are very rare.

Dilatation of the aorta is mostly located at the level of the sinuses of Valsalva, and usually is symmetrical (Fig. 3.3). In some aetiologies (*ACTA2*, *MYH11*), dilatation can also be observed in the tubular portion of the ascending aorta.

Bicuspid Aortic Valve

Some TAA have been associated with a bicuspid aortic valve (BAV), consequently the frequency of TAA is greater in patients with BAV than in the general population. The reasons for this association are unclear, and 3 main hypothesis can be proposed [18]:

- Aortic root dilatation may be constitutive, i.e. not reflecting a progressive increase in diameter with time. This may be close to the abnormal aortic cusps i.e. at the level of the sinuses of Valsalva, but not above the sino-tubular junction.
- Aortic dilatation may be secondary to a primitive alteration in the aortic wall. In fact, the histological aspect of the aortic wall of TAA-operated patients with BAV is similar to that seen in patients with Marfan syndrome or other genetic forms of TAA.
- Aortic dilatation results from alteration in the aortic flow pattern within the ascending aorta. The jet lesion historically proposed in patients with aortic stenosis has evolved into alterations in the normally laminar flow pattern of the

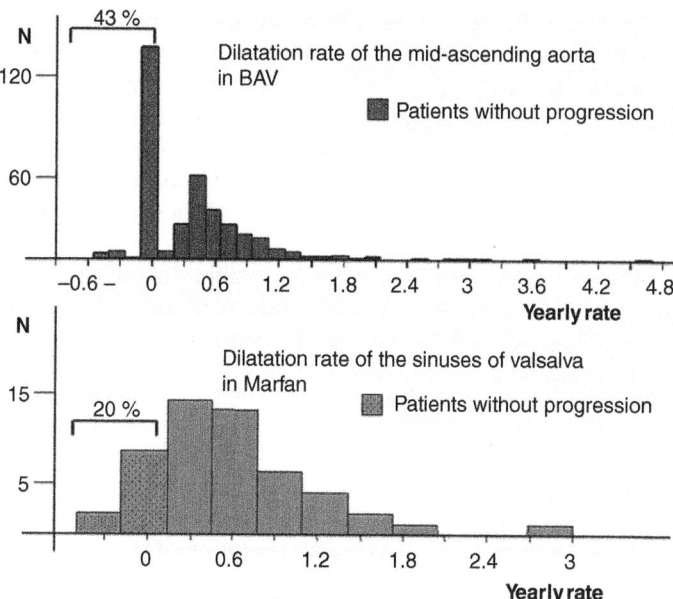

FIGURE 3.4 Aortic dilatation rate in patients with BAV and Marfan Syndrome [20]

ascending aorta, which is turbulent within the ascending aorta owing to anatomical abnormalities.

Maximum aortic diameter of TAA associated with BAV can either be localized at the level of the sinuses of Valsalva or above the sino-tubular junction. A relationship is observed between the type of the BAV and the anatomy of the aortic root: the antero-posterior diameter is increased when the BAV is related to a raphe between the two coronary artery cusps, type I R-L [19], and the aortic root progression rate is slow at the level of the sinuses of Valsalva [20]. In contrast, the dilatation of the aorta observed at the level of the tubular aorta is independent of the type of BAV and the dilatation rate is greater, which suggests that it may reflect alterations in the aortic wall and require specific care [20]. Indeed, when the dilatation rate of a population with BAV is studied, two groups are observed: patients who do not dilate over time, and those who do (Fig. 3.4).

BAV can be associated with TAA and coarctation of the aorta. Familial forms exist, but with variability (one family member present aortic dilatation whereas a second may present BAV and a third aortic dilatation and another BAV without aortic dilatation). This requires familial screening to be systematic when a BAV is observed [21]. However, no genetic defect has been clearly associated with BAV besides NOTCH1 mutation very seldom.

Given the diverse anatomy [19], embryology [22], inconstant association with aortic dilatation [20], and the presence of both familial and sporadic forms, various mechanisms may be responsible for aortic dilatation.

Turner

Women with Turner syndrome in whom aortic dilatation can also be associated with BAV and coarctation of the aorta form a specific subgroup. In these small-statured women normalization of aortic diameter is essential since the absolute diameter may under-evaluate the aortic dilatation [23]. Aortic dilatation in patients with Turner syndrome has been reported to occur in up to 40 % of cases. In this population, special care should be taken in cases of pregnancy, which is generally considered to be contraindicated in women with aortic dilatation, BAV and/or coarctation [24]. Complete imaging of the aorta (MRI or CT scanner) are necessary in these women. Patients with an index >2 cm/m^2 in the ascending aorta should be followed yearly as the risk for aortic dissection increases.

Others

Other aneurysms are neither related to any known mutation nor associated with BAV, and can be observed as sporadic or familial diseases. When familial, they are usually transmitted with a autosomal dominant pattern, and intensive research is ongoing to identify new genes involved. When sporadic, which is by far the more frequent form, the predisposing factors are usually haemodynamic (hypertension), and patient age is usually around 70.

Some specific aetiologies are seldom responsible for TAA, and are usually found in specific context: these are inflammatory diseases (see Chap. 2) (Giant cell arteritis, Takayasu disease, Kawasaki disease, Behcet Syndrome, aortitis associated with HLAB27...), or infectious diseases (Syphilis, Aspergillus, bacterial aortitis...). Obviously, when an active process responsible for aortic dilatation (such as infection) is ongoing, its treatment is warranted; however, aortic dilatation is sometimes observed years after the inflammatory phase of the disease, at a time when all therapy has long been stopped.

Descending Aorta Aneurysms

In contrast to aneurysms of the ascending aorta, aneurysms of the descending aorta are similar to aneurysms of the abdominal aorta from an epidemiological and pathophysiological point of view. Familial aggregation is present but genetic transmission is unproven and association with risk factors for atherosclerosis is the rule. In these cases, aortic dilatation is usually diffuse and not limited to a specific section. Calcification of the aortic wall is often observed. In these patients, it is obviously important to limit the risk factors.

A specific situation is the dilatation that can be observed at the initial part of the descending aorta, just below left subclavian artery level, often observed in patients with BAV and/or aortic coarctation. This dilatation appears to be present very early in life and its significance is unclear, although of the descending aorta dissections have been reported in patients with BAV [25].

Pathophysiology

TAA of the Ascending Aorta

Ascending aorta pathologies are chronic aneurismal diseases, corresponding to a progressive dilatation of the aorta, leading finally to rupture, and/or acute dissection corresponding to an intra-parietal rupture. These two pathologies are related to a progressive (aneurysms) or acute (dissections) degradation of the insoluble extracellular matrix proteins of the arterial wall, mainly elastin and collagens, which give the solidity to the arterial wall. This degradation is the fact of specific medial areas of mucoid degeneration (also formerly misnamed cystic medial necrosis), characterised by the local enrichment of alcianophilic glycosaminoglycans, vacuoles corresponding to the disappearance of smooth muscle cells, and local degradation of extracellular proteins, including disorganised adhesive proteins such as fibronectin and fibrillin and the rupture of insoluble elastin and collagen. The pathology of aneurysm and/or dissection does not differ in genetic or non-genetic aetiologies. They only clinically appear in younger patients as degenerative forms.

Role of Proteases

Fibrillin is not directly a component of the insoluble extracellular matrix of the arterial wall. Elastin and collagens are the main insoluble and hydrophobic components of the wall, giving it a strong support for resisting blood pressure (elementary contention function). Elastin is involved in wall elasticity, and is the main structural component of resistance to dilatation. Collagen is the main structural component of resistance to rupture. Both pathologies are linked to the proteolytic degradation of elastin (aneurysm) and collagen (dissection and rupture). Therefore, there is a tremendous interest in defining the panel of proteases involved in extracellular matrix degradation in Marfan syndrome and related diseases. The abundance and activity of Matrix metalloproteinases (MMPs) have been shown to be related to TAA formation in numerous studies [26]. Matrix metalloproteinase-2 is produced in mesenchymal cells; MMP-9 is produced in macrophages. We have identified the MMP-7 (matrilysin) and MMP-3 (stromelysin) as MMPs preferentially localised within the areas of mucoid degeneration [27], which probably results from their particular affinity for sulfated glycosaminoglycans.

In contrast, the data concerning serine protease activities present in aneurysm are scarce. We reported the presence of thrombin within the areas of mucoid degeneration, due, once again, to its affinity for glysosaminoglycans [28]. Interestingly enough, we recently explored the role of the plasminergic system in aneurysms of the ascending aorta, including Marfan [29]. Beside the activation of plasminogen after its binding to fibrin (fibrinolytic system), plasminogen could be activated by the plasminogen activators (PAs) expressed by mesenchymal cells. Activated plasmin released by the inter-action between plasminogen and cell-derived PAs, catalysed by membrane proteins, lead to fibronectin degradation, cell detachment [30] and apoptosis [31]. On the other hand, plas-min is able to activate MMPs, to degrade adhesive fibronectin and fibrillin, etc. and therefore to provoke the release and activation of TGF-beta of its matrix storage sites. We reported that plasminogen is transferred better from plasma to an aneurismal wall than to a normal aortic wall, that t-PA and u-PA are more expressed in an aneurismal wall than in a normal one, and therefore that generation of plasmin is enhanced in aneurismal walls as compared to normal walls, leading to an increase in TGF-beta bioavailability [29] in aneurysm of the ascending aorta. Since plasmin generation could participate to cell disappearance, MMP activation, and TGF-beta release, the fibrinolytic system is probably an important target for preventing dilatation [32]. In parallel, plasmin is also involved in dissecting pathology. In particular circulating plasmin-antiplasmin complex and fibrin degrada-tion product have been proposed as markers of acute dissec-tion, but this is probably due to the fibrinolysis of the clot in the false channel [33]. Nevertheless the participation of tissue plasmin is not excluded.

Role of TGF-Beta

In a mouse model KI for a FBN1 mutation [34], aortic dilata-tion occurs in heterozygous mice, and increased P-Smad 2 (the intracellular effecter for TGFB2) was observed in the aortic wall of pathologic mice compared to normal mice [34]. TGF-β neutralising antibodies were able to decrease the level of P-Smad 2 within the aortic wall. Besides, blocking the TGF-β pathway by the use of specific antibodies prevented abnormal aortic dilatation in this model. The idea has therefore emerged that the increased TGF-β pathway was responsible for the main anomalies associated with Marfan syndrome, rather than an abnormal structural protein directly leading to weakening of the extracellular matrix and tissues.

However, TGF-beta 1 activates both Smad and non-Smad pathways, and we were not able to find any activation of these non-Smad pathways in the aortic wall of patients with Marfan syndrome, nor were we able to find increased mRNA levels for TGF-beta 1 within the aortic wall [35]. This was true for the aortic walls of patients with Marfan syndrome as well as for aortic walls from patients with aortic aneurysms from other aetiologies (bicuspid aortic valve, non syndromic TAA).

In contrast, we were able to demonstrate an increase in P-Smad 2 in smooth muscle cells from the aortic wall of patients with Marfan syndrome but also patients with thoracic aortic aneurysms from other aetiologies [35]. Actually, we and others have also reported increased P-Smad-2 in the aortic wall of patients with TAA secondary to mutation in the TGF-β receptor, despite the fact that the mutation in the TGF-β receptor alters (blocks) the transmission of the signal [9, 36]; this suggests that increased Psmad-2 within the aortic wall is not secondary to increased TGF-β activation in human aorta. Beside, no clear association in localisation could be found between the Smad 2 nuclear levels and the TGF-β extracellular staining in the aortic wall of patients with aneurysmal aorta, also suggesting the absence of a direct link between the two observations [35].

All this data questions the simple cause and effect relationship that has been proposed between TGF-β activation and aortic root dilatation in Marfan syndrome, but widens the potential importance of the TGF-β pathway alteration in the aortic aneurysm disease: it suggests that actually, increased Smad-2 within the aortic wall is related to a "common pathway" observed in all forms of TAA, which could either be responsible for (as suggested by the beneficial effect of neutralising antibodies) or responsive to (as would have been anticipated by the known pro-fibrotic and anti-proteolytic effects of TGF-β) the dilatation of the aorta. This last hypothesis is also compatible with the correlation observed between increased Smad-2 level and the degree of elastic fibre fragmentation that we observed in aortic aneurismal wall of diverse aetiologies [35].

Dissociation between TGF-β activation and increase in Smad-2 signalling was further supported by recent experiments from our group. We were able to demonstrate that (1) increased P-Smad-2 was specific to smooth muscle cell (SMC) i.e. not present in fibroblasts obtained from the aortic wall despite the fact that all cells should be submitted to the same TGF-β stimulation coming from the extracellular matrix within the same aortic wall, (2) increased P-Smad-2 was associated with increased Smad-2 RNA level within SMC (which was not present in the fibroblasts coming from the same aortic wall) (3) this deregulation of the Smad 2 pathway within the SMC was heritable, i.e. increased P-Smad 2 concentration was maintained during SMC culture, despite the absence of TGF-β within the culture milieu [37], indicating an epigenetic control of increased Smad-2 within the SMC. Actually this epigenetic control was further suggested by chromatin immuno-precipitation, showing alterations of the histones linked to the promoter of the Smad-2 gene within the SMC [37]. These observations were made in cells derived from aneurismal aortic wall from various aetiologies (i.e. patients with Marfan syndrome but also patients with aortic aneurysms from other aetiologies) compared to SMC derived from normal human aorta.

As a conclusion regarding these observations, we can say that increased P-Smad-2 within the SMC of aortic aneurismal wall is observed whatever the aetiology of the aneurysm, and that its relation to TGF-β activation is not clearly established. Actually, this may be a compensatory mechanism induced within the smooth muscle cell of aneurismal wall independent from the aetiology of the aneurysm.

This discussion is of importance the interpretation of the beneficial effect of losartan if proven, because this mechanism should determine which is the population that could benefit from this therapy: only Marfan patients or all patients with TAA (see below for discussion)

Imaging Follow-up and Risk of Complications

A patient with a TAA should be followed-up by a cardiologist, and have regular imaging of the aorta. It is usually recommended that TTE should be repeated after 6 months to ensure the absence of rapid evolution of the aortic dilatation when a TAA is recognized for the first time in a patient [21, 38]. Thereafter a yearly imaging is considered sufficient, unless the aortic diameter is coming close to the surgical threshold. Then echocardiography every 6 months may be wise [38]. Diameter expansion, severity of aortic regurgitation, and left ventricular function may be correctly evaluated when the echocardiographic window is adequate.

Echocardiography does not allow visualization of the entire aorta. Therefore, the use of MRI or CT scanner to obtain complete imaging of the aorta is recommended when the TAA is first recognized for two reasons: first validation of the aortic diameter measure obtained with echocardiography, which will be used during follow-up; second being able to confirm future increase in aortic diameter evidenced with echocardiography. This is recommended because of the variability of the aortic measure and the limited increase in aortic diameter felt to be significant [38].

Aneurysms of arteries others than the aorta can be observed in some genetic TAA such as those secondary to mutations in genes coding for proteins of the TGF-B pathway (*TGFB2*, *TGFBR1*, *TGFBR2*, *SMAD3*). Visualization of all the arteries is then necessary during the initial evaluation of the patient, including cerebral arteries, either using CT scanner, or MRI. How often these imaging should be repeated remains speculative, no general rules can be proposed at the present time. These patients should be taken care off by cardiologist interested in these diseases, and the decision made on a case by case basis.

Surgery

Aortic size is the principal predictor of aortic rupture or dissection. The risk of rupture or dissection of thoracic aortic aneurysms increases significantly when the aorta size is greater than 60 mm [39]. The growth rate of an aneurysm depends on its aetiology: a rate of 0.5 mm/year is reported for TAA of the ascending aorta of genetic origin (mutation *FBN1*), a similar rate in patients with TAA and BAV and a much lower rate in patients with isolated TAA occurring with tricuspid aortic valve and no familial history [20]. This is reflected by the age at which these different groups are proposed for surgery (Fig. 3.1) and is rendering accurate measurements of change [40] and clinical trials challenging. The dissection and rupture rates of TAAs are also dependent on aneurysm site (ascending or descending aorta). In the ascending aorta, a steep increase in complication rates is observed once the aneurysm exceeds 60 mm in diameter as shown by the retrospective study from Yale [39]. Above that diameter, the rate of aortic dissection and rupture increases to 30 % a year. In descending aortic aneurysms (including aneurysms on chronic aortic dissection), this occurs when the diameter reaches 70 mm. The 5-year survival rate from untreated TAAs has been reported to be between 19 [41] and 64 % [42, 43].

Surgery is usually indicated for an aortic diameter ≥50 mm in Marfan syndrome, decreasing to 45 mm in the presence of risk factors such as rapid increase in aortic diameter (>3 mm), family history of dissection and hypertension [38]. For the other genetic TAA, case-by-case evaluation is necessary, since the natural history of these newly recognized diseases is not well established and reports contradictory, probably because of different population recruitments in different studies [9, 12].

In the case of BAV, surgery is proposed for a diameter of ≥55 mm, unless risk factors such as hypertension, history of dissection, aortic coarctation are present, lowering the threshold to 50 mm [38]. Finally, when no BAV or family history is present, surgery is proposed for an aortic diameter ≥55 mm.

Recommendations which can be made are less clear for the descending aorta: the indication is largely dependent on the risk associated with the surgery itself, which is varying with the location of the aneurysm (only thoracic vs. thoraco-abdominal), the choice to replace only the thoracic descending aorta or the thoraco-abdominal aorta (which is associated with greater mortality and more difficult postoperative course), the other risk factors of the patients (including pulmonary and renal diseases), the presence of a degenerative underlying genetic aortic disease and its type, the extend of the dissected aorta. Indication for intervening may also be influenced by the possibility of endovascular stenting which is associated with lower per procedure complications but is not accepted in patients with a genetic aortic disease.

Lifestyle

Because the aortic dilatation is reflecting weakness of the aortic wall and beneficial therapy is limiting the stress applied to the aortic wall, one would logically propose to limit aortic stress induced by exercise in this population: during strenuous exercise, a rise in aortic pressure is observed which can be very important in isometric sports (>300 mmHg [44]). There is actually no trial showing the beneficial effect of sport limitation in this population, but few case reports of aortic dissection occurring during exercise in young patients. The classification of sports usually used is that of Mitchell (Fig. 3.5), reporting the Bethesda conference in 2005 [45]. No rules have been established beyond that proposed for patients with Marfan syndrome [46, 47], but one can extrapolate to patients with other genetic defects, and probably with patients presenting TAA of other etiologies. There, the restriction is probably to be balanced by

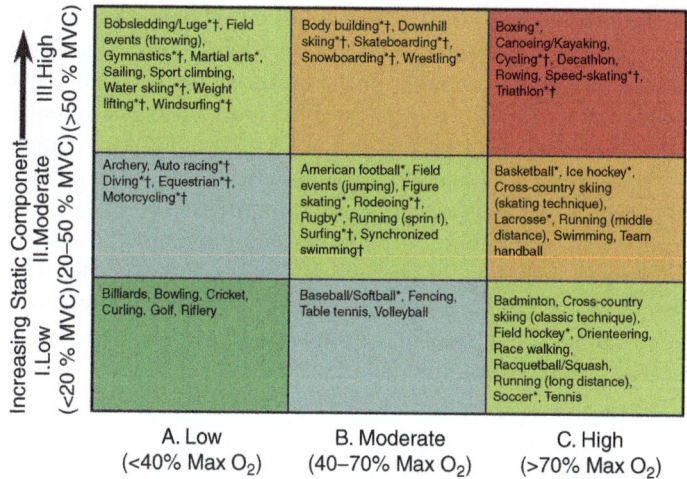

FIGURE 3.5 Classification of sports [45]. *Danger of bodily collision. †Increased risk if syncope occurs

the evolution profile of the patient (i.e. the precise pathology he presents, association or not with BAV, location of the dilatation, history of the patient and of his family).

Besides, the tachycardia also increases the stress applied to the aortic wall, and this should be limited by the β-blocker therapy.

Pharmacotherapy for TAA of the Ascending Aorta

Therapy Aimed at Limiting the Haemodynamic Stress Imposed on the Aortic Wall

The goals of medical therapy have traditionally been to reduce shear stress on the aneurysmal segment of the aorta by reducing blood pressure and contractility (dP/dt). The understanding that aortic dilatation is favored by intraluminal pressure within the aorta, the repetitive distension with the systolic ejection, has led to the proposal of therapies aimed at limiting these factors in patients with thoracic aortic aneurysms. Indeed, the proof of concept have been obtained in a population "pure" for the presence of TAA, i.e. population of patient with TAA of genetic origin, Marfan patients. These studies are reported in the chapter on Marfan syndrome. In short β-blocker therapy slows aortic root dilatation in an unblinded randomized study including 70 patients older than 12 years [48], and retrospective studies indicate similar benefit in children [49]. Losartan has been shown in a randomized study to reduce the aortic root dilatation rate in adults [50].

Therapy Aimed at Acting on the Biological Mechanisms of Aortic Dilatation

TAA of Genetic Origin

We discussed the observation of increased P-Smad2 in the aortic wall made in the mouse model KI for a *FBN1* mutation, and the beneficial effect of TGF-β antibodies, suggesting that the activation of the TGF-beta pathway was actually responsible for the dilatation of the aorta in Marfan Syndrome [34]. In the same study, mice were given high dose of losartan during growth, which resulted in limitation (even complete prevention) of aortic dilatation in the animals. Simultaneously, P-Smad2 was decreased in the aortic wall of the mouse, which was interpreted as the demonstration that losartan limited aortic dilatation through blockade of the TGF-β pathway, which was responsible for the beneficial effect of the drug. Blocking the biological mechanism responsible for aortic dilatation would be ideal. However it is debated whether activation of the TGF-β pathway (as indicated by the increased P-Smad2) is causative for aortic dilatation or only secondary to aortic dilatation, because P-Smad2 was found to be increased within the aortic wall of patients with aortic aneurysm regardless the aetiology of the aneurysm (including

TAA associated with BAV or sporadic forms), not only in the aortic wall of patients with TAA secondary to mutation in the *FBN1* gene [35]. This suggests that the increased P-Smad2 is an adaptive phenomenon observed during the development of aortic dilatation and therefore just a marker of the alteration of the aortic wall. This marker is increasing with increasing dilatation and decreasing in the absence of dilatation as expected for a marker. This view is also in line with the recent results in the mouse model KI for a mutation in the *TGFBR2* gene, in which TGFB antibodies were not able to limit or prevent aortic dilatation, in contrast to what was reported in the *FBN1* KI mouse model [51]. Despite this opposite finding, losartan was efficacious in the TGFBR2 model for limiting or preventing aortic dilatation in the animals, as it was in the FBN1 mouse model.

Losartan is usually known and used for its vasodilatory effect secondary to the blockade of the renin-angiotensin-aldosteron axis, and indicated as such for hypertension and heart failure. The beneficial effect of this drug in the mouse with a *FBN1* gene mutation (which has been reproduced by different teams) could then be the result of its haemodynamic effect, limiting the rebound wave and therefore limiting the systolic aortic pressure within the aortic root.

The importance of central systolic arterial pressure has been highlighted in multiple studies. In studies on hypertension (LIFE study [52–54]), the comparison of β-blocker with losartan demonstrated better outcome in patients receiving losartan compared to patients receiving atenolol, whereas the mean decrease in blood pressure was similar. A proposed explanation was that the decrease in systolic blood pressure in the central aorta differed between the two groups, being lower in those receiving losartan owing to the limitation of the rebound wave, a consequence of the vasodilatation induced by the drug. Central systolic blood pressure is actually the afterload imposed on the left ventricle, and its decrease was associated with a greater reduction in left ventricular mass in patients receiving losartan. Similarly, we showed the systolic blood pressure in the ascending aorta to be a major determinant of aortic dilatation in patients with aortic aneurysm related to Marfan syndrome [55]. It is therefore highly likely that the beneficial effect observed in the mouse model is related to lower central pressure in the animal.

Whatever the mechanism responsible for the beneficial effect of losartan observed in the mouse model was, this observation has led to the launching of multiple clinical trials, which are reported in the Marfan chapter of this book. Some compare losartan with placebo, others losartan with beta-blockade, others irbesartan with a β-blocker or a combination of the two drugs. Most are ongoing, or just closed, and the first reported results seem to indicate a beneficial effect [50].

What is the similarity of the Marfan and the non Marfan population? In the present chapter focused on TAA not related to Marfan syndrome, the key issue is the applicability of the potentially positive results of the Sartan trials conducted only in patients with Marfan Syndrome in the non Marfan population. The answer to this central question is secondary to the understanding of two mechanisms: (1) the fact that the aortic dilatation observed when a genetic abnormality is present reflects imperfection of the repair process of the aortic wall after physiological aggression during life (2) the mechanism of action of losartan.

One can consider that the extra-cellular matrix, the TGFB pathway and the smooth muscle cells contractile apparatus are all involved in the dilatation process. The dilatation is only the result of imperfect repair of the aortic wall after an aggression: aortic blood pressure and systolic distension of the aorta tend to dilate the aorta. Normally during life, aortic wall faces this aggression, and the extracellular matrix, the TGFB pathway and the smooth muscle cell contractile apparatus are all involved in the repair process of the aortic wall. The progressive increase in the aortic diameter with aging in the general normal population illustrates the existence and the "normality" of this aggression and the existence of the secondary repair: aortic remodeling is a physiological phenomenon during life in the general population even in the absence of mutation in one of the genes cited earlier, and the aortic wall is a biological tissue including living cells and not only a passive container. The rapid (0.5 mm/year) dilatation of the aorta in the Marfan population or in patients with TAA from other etiologies (0.5 mm/year in patients with BAV, slower in sporadic forms in elderly patients [20]) can then be viewed as the consequence of the lesser complete repair of the aortic wall in patients carrying a mutation in a gene involved in the reparation process. This is intuitively acceptable for mutations in genes coding for extracellular matrix proteins (such as FBN1) or genes involved in the fibrosis processes (such as genes involved in the TGF-beta pathway) and may be true for genes altering the ability of the smooth muscle cell to react to aggression (such as genes coding for the contractile apparatus of the smooth muscle cell) because of the alteration of the proper perception of extracellular milieu as a consequence of these mutations [56]: when one of the processes involved in the repair is deficient, then the imperfection of the repair increases meaning increased aortic dilatation rate, and the aortic aneurysm can occur. In other words, whatever the etiology of the aneurysms, the pathophysiology is probably similar, so that a therapy effective within a group of patient will probably also be effective in another group of patients with TAA. Thus, losartan should be beneficial in all patients with TAA, whatever the etiology even if its mechanism of action is supposed not to be mediated through its hemodynamic effects.

If one believes that the benefit of losartan is the result of a diminished stress applied to the aortic wall, i.e. the consequence of its vasodilatory effect, then the applicability of the results obtained in the whole population carrying a TAA is even more logical.

The conclusion of this long reasoning is therefore that a therapy which is efficacious in a group of patients with TAA should be beneficial in all the patients with TAA. Of course, this conclusion cannot be established with certainty in the absence of randomized trial (evidence based medicine), but the probability that such a clinical trial be soon available remains low. Some trials are ongoing trying to evaluate the benefit of sartan in population different from Marfan: the BAV Study (Beta Blockers and Angiotensin Receptor Blockers in Bicuspid Aortic Valve Disease Aortopathy [BAV Study NCT01202721]) is recruiting patients with BAV in Canada and will compare the rate of ascending aortic growth by magnetic resonance imaging in patients randomized to ARB therapy (telmisartan) versus betablocker (atenolol) versus placebo in 416 patients. This study started in June 2011, and is supposed to finish by July 2016. Another study from University of Michigan is looking for intermediate markers (MMP plasma levels) and aortic dilatation in patients with BAV (NCT01390181).

It is also unknown if the benefit of ACEI would be similar to that of the Sartan, with conflicting results in animals and positive retrospective studies in humans with MFS.

Practical Considerations

In a patient with TAA, the practical issues are twofold: should the patient be treated, and if yes, which drug should be used?

Should the Patient Be Medically Treated?

The answer to this question is the result of a balance between risk and benefit.

The risk of the disease is its progression, since when it is feared that the risk is rupture, the treatment is surgery. The risk of progression is greater when aortic dilatation is observed in a young patient, or when the history of the patient reports progression over the last years. The etiology of the TAA is also an important factor, as the presence of a genetic factor, either identified or suspected because of the familial history, indicates that the underlying defect responsible for the dilatation of the aorta is a permanent one. Therefore, the indication for medical therapy is wide. It is accompanied by the limitation of physically demanding violent sports, and the exclusion of competitive sports, with the aim of limiting the increase in the aortic pressure secondary to theses intensive activities.

Which Drug Should Be Used?

The risk of therapy is low, but the tolerance may not be perfect. The first line therapy is usually a β-blocker, because we have a randomized study in the Marfan population [48]. The β-blocker used in this study was propranolol, but the beta-blockers used nowadays in this indication are not limited to propranolol. There is a theoretical advantage in using a vasodilatory beta-blocker owing to limitation of the rebound wave, and therefore the decrease in the central systolic blood pressure; however, no clinical study has been performed to date to demonstrate this hypothesis. Since a decrease of heart rate is thought to be the main beneficial effect of β-blockers in this population, the use of molecules devoid of agonist effect is favoured. The legitimacy of giving β-blocker to patients with aortic fragility not related to mutation in *FBN1* is reinforced by the results of BESTT, which evaluated bucindolol in patients with vascular Ehlers Danlos; in this disease related to mutation in *Col3A1*, the aorta is more prone to dissection than dilatation, and the fragility of the vessels is also observed in medium sized arteries. Bucindolol was able to decrease the rate of clinical event in this disease [57].

When the tolerance of the beta-blocker is not good, the attitude can be (1) to decrease the dosage because of excessive bradycardia (2) try another beta-blocker with different pharmacological properties (3) change the beta-blocker for a drug with similar hemodynamic action, i.c. a calcium blocker, such as verapamil or isoptine. These drugs have been shown in retrospective studies performed in children to lower the rate of aortic dilatation [49], (4) propose losartan for theoretical consideration, the mouse model, and preliminary positive results in humans [50]. The dosage should be 100 mg/day, and the question remains whether we should stick to this molecule or whether all sartans are similar for this purpose. If one considers that the main effect is an hemodynamic effect, then an ACEI can also be proposed [58]. One may wonder how ivabradine would behave in this situation [59].

Whatever the drug proposed, it must be borne in mind that this is going to be a lifelong treatment, or at least a treatment to continue until surgery is performed if this occurs, in a patient without any complains or limitation due to the disease. It therefore has to be well tolerated, and the tolerance/benefit risk should be evaluated individually.

Is Medical Therapy Useful After Surgery?

When the dilated part of the ascending aorta has been replaced, the question arises as whether there is any reason for pursuing medical therapy aiming at protecting the aorta. The response is dependent on the fact that the remaining aorta is or is not susceptible to dilatation, in other word dependant on the extent of the abnormality along the aorta. Usually, the presence of a mutation in a gene responsible for TAA indicates a risk for aortic dilatation or dissection beyond the ascending aorta, and therefore indicates that medical therapy should be prolonged after surgery.

When no genetic factors can be recognized, the answer is more difficult: the group of patients with TAA in relation with bicuspid aortic valve is heterogeneous, with aortic dilatation which can occur only at the level of the sinuses of Valsalva, or only at the ascending aorta, but can also sometimes on the aortic arch, and on the initial part of the descending aorta [60]. Moreover, reports of patients with bicuspid aortic valve presenting dissection of the descending aorta also suggest that the fragility of the aortic wall can go beyond the ascending aorta [25]. Therefore, it is logical to continue therapy after surgery in this population if it is well tolerated and not limiting for the patient.

When an older patient is operated on because of ascending TAA, the presence of other risk factors usually renders the treatment of hypertension necessary, and therefore the treatment is pursued; however, when the aortic dilatation is limited to the part which has been replaced, and the patient present no risk factors requiring treatment, it may be logical to limit care to repeated and regular follow-up.

Pharmacotherapy for TAA
of the Descending Aorta

Treatment Aimed at Limiting the Atherosclerosis Process Responsible for Dilatation of the Descending Aorta

The descending part of the thoracic aorta is more prone to diseases similar to that of the abdominal aorta, i.e. atherosclerosis. Atherosclerosis is a diffuse disease, and factors limiting the development of atherosclerosis should therefore be beneficial for patients with TAA of the descending aorta beyond their effect on the abdominal aorta. Besides, the aorta is prone to dilate, rupture, but may also be responsible for embolic events in the branches of the aorta (notably the renal arteries, and the arteries of the legs). Actually, data on the benefit of medical therapy in patients with abdominal aortic aneurysm is limited: β-blocker therapy have given contradictory results [61–63], similar to ACEI [64, 65]. Since the etiology is atherosclerosis, the therapy should include aspirin, and active treatment of risk factors; smoking is particularly harmful, hypertension should be perfectly controlled, and statins should be the rule.

In recent years stress has been put on the importance of dental hygiene because of the responsibility of periodontal infection in the colonization of the thrombus with germs which are favoring aortic dilatation, e.g. porphyromonas gingivalis [66], which could in part explain benefit reported with antibiotics in AAA.

Therapies to Be Tested for Tomorrow

MMP Inhibitors

Since matrix metalloproteinase (MMP), i.e. enzyme that degrades protein within the extra-cellular, and need Zinc as a cofactor) have to be involved in aortic remodeling, MMP inhibitors are expected to limit aortic dilatation. Aortic dilatation can only occur if proteolysis occurs in the aortic wall, allowing replacement by new molecules arranged differently so as to get a greater aortic diameter; MMP have to be implicated in this process. Actually increase in MMP plasma levels have been reported in aortic aneurismal patients. Study of aortic wall of patients operated on for TAA have reported increased RNA levels of MMP suggesting also their role in aortic dilatation [67]. Increased MMP activity have also been reported [68], and we reported direct visualization of MMP 3 and 7 within the aortic wall of TAA [29].

Doxycycline is a non-specific MMP inhibitor which has been used in humans as an antibiotic (macrolide). There is very limited indication that this drug may reduce aortic dilatation in humans, but there are more important data in the animals, including in the mouse model KI for *FBN1* mutation [69–71].

Statins

The use of statins in patients with TAA of the descending aorta, related to atherosclerosis, is established although direct proof of benefit is lacking. There are some indications that statins may lower the aortic dilatation rate in aneurysm related to genetic defects in the mouse model KI for the *FBN1* mutation [72].

No prospective study in human has been performed to date, but two recent retrospective analyses from the Aortic Institute at Yale-New Haven Hospital suggest a possible therapeutic benefit of statin treatment in TAA population [43]; In a retrospective study of 1,561 patients with thoracic aneurysms, statin therapy usage was associated with protection against complications of thoracic aortic aneurysms, especially those in the descending aorta, which is consistent with the importance of atherosclerosis in this group of patients, as opposed to patients with TAA of the ascending aorta, particularly of the aortic root. In patients taking statin therapy, the time to surgery and complications, including aortic dissection, rupture or death, was significantly delayed ($p < 0.001$).

Others

Fibrinolytic activity has been shown to be possible within the aortic wall [29], and could participate with the MMP in the aortic wall destruction/reconstruction process leading to aortic dilatation. Interacting with this system could therefore be associated with limited dilatation in patients with TAA.

Conclusion

The pharmacotherapy available for the treatment of thoracic aortic aneurysm is very limited, and actually derived from the studies conducted in selected populations such as patients with Marfan syndrome. In short, β-blockers remain the reference therapy, possibly with losartan as a second-line option. Limitation of physically-demanding sports is aimed at avoiding the brisk increases in blood pressure and therefore the stress imposed on the aortic wall.

Studies in patients presenting TAA of non-genetic aetiology are needed, and hopefully progress made in the understanding of their pathophysiology will transfer into efficacious medical alternatives to surgery which to date remains the therapy of choice.

References

1. Braverman AC. Medical management of thoracic aortic aneurysm disease. J Thorac Cardiovasc Surg. 2013;145(3 Suppl):S2–6.
2. Albornoz G, Coady MA, Roberts M, Davies RR, Tranquilli M, Rizzo JA, et al. Familial thoracic aortic aneurysms and dissections – incidence, modes of inheritance, and phenotypic patterns. Ann Thorac Surg. 2006;82(4):1400–5.
3. Ito S, Akutsu K, Tamori Y, Sakamoto S, Yoshimuta T, Hashimoto H, et al. Differences in atherosclerotic profiles between patients with thoracic and abdominal aortic aneurysms. Am J Cardiol. 2008;101(5):696–9.
4. Danyi P, Elefteriades JA, Jovin IS. Medical therapy of thoracic aortic aneurysms: are we there yet? Circulation. 2011;124(13):1469–76.

5. Pyeritz RE. Heritable thoracic aortic disorders. Curr Opin Cardiol. 2014;29(1):97–102.

6. De Paepe A, Devereux RB, Dietz HC, Hennekam RC, Pyeritz RE. Revised diagnostic criteria for the Marfan syndrome. Am J Med Genet. 1996;62(4):417–26.

7. Loeys BL, Dietz HC, Braverman AC, Callewaert BL, De Backer J, Devereux RB, et al. The revised Ghent nosology for the Marfan syndrome. J Med Genet. 2010;47(7):476–85.

8. Pope FM, Narcisi P, Nicholls AC, Germaine D, Pals G, Richards AJ. COL3A1 mutations cause variable clinical phenotypes including acrogeria and vascular rupture. Br J Dermatol. 1996; 135(2):163–81.

9. Loeys BL, Schwarze U, Holm T, Callewaert BL, Thomas GH, Pannu H, et al. Aneurysm syndromes caused by mutations in the TGF-beta receptor. N Engl J Med. 2006;355(8):788–98.

10. Loeys BL, Chen J, Neptune ER, Judge DP, Podowski M, Holm T, et al. A syndrome of altered cardiovascular, craniofacial, neuro-cognitive and skeletal development caused by mutations in TGFBR1 or TGFBR2. Nat Genet. 2005;37(3):275–81.

11. Pannu H, Fadulu VT, Chang J, Lafont A, Hasham SN, Sparks E, et al. Mutations in transforming growth factor-beta receptor type II cause familial thoracic aortic aneurysms and dissections. Circulation. 2005;112(4):513–20.

12. Attias D, Stheneur C, Roy C, Collod-Beroud G, Detaint D, Faivre L, et al. Comparison of clinical presentations and outcomes between patients with TGFBR2 and FBN1 mutations in Marfan syndrome and related disorders. Circulation. 2009;120(25):2541–9.

13. Aubart M, Gobert D, Aubart-Cohen F, Detaint D, Hanna N, d'Indya H, et al. Early-onset osteoarthritis, charcot-marie-tooth like neuropathy, autoimmune features, multiple arterial aneu-rysms and dissections: an unrecognized and life threatening condition. PLoS One. 2014;9(5):e96387.

14. Boileau C, Guo DC, Hanna N, Regalado ES, Detaint D, Gong L, et al. TGFB2 mutations cause familial thoracic aortic aneurysms and dissections associated with mild systemic features of Marfan syndrome. Nat Genet. 2012;44(8):916–21.

15. Guo DC, Pannu H, Tran-Fadulu V, Papke CL, Yu RK, Avidan N, et al. Mutations in smooth muscle alpha-actin (ACTA2) lead to thoracic aortic aneurysms and dissections. Nat Genet. 2007;39(12):1488–93.

16. Guo DC, Papke CL, Tran-Fadulu V, Regalado ES, Avidan N, Johnson RJ, et al. Mutations in smooth muscle alpha-actin

(ACTA2) cause coronary artery disease, stroke, and Moyamoya disease, along with thoracic aortic disease. Am J Hum Genet. 2009;84(5):617–27.

17. Zhu L, Vranckx R, Khau Van Kien P, Lalande A, Boisset N, Mathieu F, et al. Mutations in myosin heavy chain 11 cause a syndrome associating thoracic aortic aneurysm/aortic dissection and patent ductus arteriosus. Nat Genet. 2006;38(3):343–9.

18. Sievers HH, Sievers HL. Aortopathy in bicuspid aortic valve disease – genes or hemodynamics? or Scylla and Charybdis? Eur J Cardiothorac Surg. 2011;39(6):803–4.

19. Sievers HH, Schmidtke C. A classification system for the bicuspid aortic valve from 304 surgical specimens. J Thorac Cardiovasc Surg. 2007;133(5):1226–33.

20. Detaint D, Michelena HI, Nkomo VT, Vahanian A, Jondeau G, Sarano ME. Aortic dilatation patterns and rates in adults with bicuspid aortic valves: a comparative study with Marfan syndrome and degenerative aortopathy. Heart. 2014;100(2):126–34.

21. Hiratzka LF, Bakris GL, Beckman JA, Bersin RM, Carr VF, Casey Jr DE, et al. 2010 ACCF/AHA/AATS/ACR/ASA/SCA/SCAI/SIR/STS/SVM guidelines for the diagnosis and management of patients with Thoracic Aortic Disease: a report of the American College of Cardiology Foundation/American Heart Association Task Force on Practice Guidelines, American Association for Thoracic Surgery, American College of Radiology, American Stroke Association, Society of Cardiovascular Anesthesiologists, Society for Cardiovascular Angiography and Interventions, Society of Interventional Radiology, Society of Thoracic Surgeons, and Society for Vascular Medicine. Circulation. 2010;121(13):e266–369.

22. Fernandez B, Duran AC, Fernandez-Gallego T, Fernandez MC, Such M, Arque JM, et al. Bicuspid aortic valves with different spatial orientations of the leaflets are distinct etiological entities. J Am Coll Cardiol. 2009;54(24):2312–8.

23. Matura LA, Ho VB, Rosing DR, Bondy CA. Aortic dilatation and dissection in Turner syndrome. Circulation. 2007;116(15):1663–70.

24. Cabanes L, Chalas C, Christin-Maitre S, Donadille B, Felten ML, Gaxotte V, et al. Turner syndrome and pregnancy: clinical practice. Recommendations for the management of patients with Turner syndrome before and during pregnancy. Eur J Obstet Gynecol Reprod Biol. 2010;152(1):18–24.

25. Michelena HI, Khanna AD, Mahoney D, Margaryan E, Topilsky Y, Suri RM, et al. Incidence of aortic complications in patients with bicuspid aortic valves. JAMA. 2011;306(10):1104–12.

26. Barbour JR, Spinale FG, Ikonomidis JS. Proteinase systems and thoracic aortic aneurysm progression. J Surg Res. 2007;139(2): 292–307.

27. Borges LF, Touat Z, Leclercq A, Zen AA, Jondeau G, Franc B, et al. Tissue diffusion and retention of metalloproteinases in ascending aortic aneurysms and dissections. Hum Pathol. 2009;40(3):306–13.

28. Touat Z, Lepage L, Ollivier V, Nataf P, Hvass U, Labreuche J, et al. Dilation-dependent activation of platelets and prothrombin in human thoracic ascending aortic aneurysm. Arterioscler Thromb Vasc Biol. 2008;28(5):940–6.

29. Borges LF, Gomez D, Quintana M, Touat Z, Jondeau G, Leclercq A, et al. Fibrinolytic activity is associated with presence of cystic medial degeneration in aneurysms of the ascending aorta. Histopathology. 2010;57(6):917–32.

30. Meilhac O, Ho-Tin-Noe B, Houard X, Philippe M, Michel JB, Angles-Cano E. Pericellular plasmin induces smooth muscle cell anoikis. FASEB J. 2003;17(10):1301–3.

31. Michel JB. Anoikis in the cardiovascular system: known and unknown extracellular mediators. Arterioscler Thromb Vasc Biol. 2003;23(12):2146–54.

32. Plow EF, Hoover-Plow J. The functions of plasminogen in cardiovascular disease. Trends Cardiovasc Med. 2004;14(5):180–6.

33. Nagaoka K, Sadamatsu K, Yamawaki T, Shikada T, Sagara S, Ohe K, et al. Fibrinogen/fibrin degradation products in acute aortic dissection. Intern Med. 2010;49(18):1943–7.

34. Habashi JP, Judge DP, Holm TM, Cohn RD, Loeys BL, Cooper TK, et al. Losartan, an AT1 antagonist, prevents aortic aneurysm in a mouse model of Marfan syndrome. Science. 2006;312(5770):117–21.

35. Gomez D, Al Haj Zen A, Borges LF, Philippe M, Gutierrez PS, Jondeau G, et al. Syndromic and non-syndromic aneurysms of the human ascending aorta share activation of the Smad2 pathway. J Pathol. 2009;218(1):131–42.

36. Mizuguchi T, Collod-Beroud G, Akiyama T, Abifadel M, Harada N, Morisaki T, et al. Heterozygous TGFBR2 mutations in Marfan syndrome. Nat Genet. 2004;36(8):855–60.

37. Gomez D, Coyet A, Ollivier V, Jeunemaitre X, Jondeau G, Michel JB, et al. Epigenetic control of vascular smooth muscle cells in Marfan and non-Marfan thoracic aortic aneurysms. Cardiovasc Res. 2011;89(2):446–56.

38. Vahanian A, Alfieri O, Andreotti F, Antunes MJ, Baron-Esquivias G, Baumgartner H, et al. Guidelines on the management of

valvular heart disease (version 2012). Eur Heart J. 2012;33(19): 2451–96.

39. Davies RR, Goldstein LJ, Coady MA, Tittle SL, Rizzo JA, Kopf GS, et al. Yearly rupture or dissection rates for thoracic aortic aneurysms: simple prediction based on size. Ann Thorac Surg. 2002;73(1):17–27; discussion –8.

40. Evangelista A. Imaging aortic aneurysmal disease. Heart. 2014;100(12):909–15.

41. Coady MA, Rizzo JA, Hammond GL, Mandapati D, Darr U, Kopf GS, et al. What is the appropriate size criterion for resection of thoracic aortic aneurysms? J Thorac Cardiovasc Surg. 1997;113(3):476–91; discussion 89–91.

42. Bickerstaff LK, Pairolero PC, Hollier LH, Melton LJ, Van Peenen HJ, Cherry KJ, et al. Thoracic aortic aneurysms: a population-based study. Surgery. 1982;92(6):1103–8.

43. Coady MA, Rizzo JA, Goldstein LJ, Elefteriades JA. Natural history, pathogenesis, and etiology of thoracic aortic aneurysms and dissections. Cardiol Clin. 1999;17(4):615–35, vii.

44. MacDougall JD, Tuxen D, Sale DG, Moroz JR, Sutton JR. Arterial blood pressure response to heavy resistance exercise. J Appl Physiol (1985). 1985;58(3):785–90.

45. Mitchell JH, Haskell W, Snell P, Van Camp SP. Task Force 8: classification of sports. J Am Coll Cardiol. 2005;45(8):1364–7.

46. Maron BJ, Ackerman MJ, Nishimura RA, Pyeritz RE, Towbin JA, Udelson JE. Task Force 4: HCM and other cardiomyopathies, mitral valve prolapse, myocarditis, and Marfan syndrome. J Am Coll Cardiol. 2005;45(8):1340–5.

47. Keane MG, Pyeritz RE. Medical management of Marfan syndrome. Circulation. 2008;117(21):2802–13.

48. Shores J, Berger KR, Murphy EA, Pyeritz RE. Progression of aortic dilatation and the benefit of long-term beta-adrenergic blockade in Marfan's syndrome. N Engl J Med. 1994;330(19):1335–41.

49. Ladouceur M, Fermanian C, Lupoglazoff JM, Edouard T, Dulac Y, Acar P, et al. Effect of beta-blockade on ascending aortic dilatation in children with the Marfan syndrome. Am J Cardiol. 2007;99(3):406–9.

50. Groenink M, den Hartog AW, Franken R, Radonic T, de Waard V, Timmermans J, et al. Losartan reduces aortic dilatation rate in adults with Marfan syndrome: a randomized controlled trial. Eur Heart J. 2013;2.

51. Gallo EM, Loch DC, Habashi JP, Calderon JF, Chen Y, Bedja D, et al. Angiotensin II-dependent TGF-beta signaling contributes

to Loeys-Dietz syndrome vascular pathogenesis. J Clin Invest. 2014;124(1):448–60.

52. Dahlof B, Devereux RB, Kjeldsen SE, Julius S, Beevers G, de Faire U, et al. Cardiovascular morbidity and mortality in the Losartan Intervention For Endpoint reduction in hypertension study (LIFE): a randomised trial against atenolol. Lancet. 2002;359(9311):995–1003.

53. Okin PM, Devereux RB, Jern S, Kjeldsen SE, Julius S, Nieminen MS, et al. Regression of electrocardiographic left ventricular hypertrophy by losartan versus atenolol: the Losartan Intervention for Endpoint reduction in Hypertension (LIFE) Study. Circulation. 2003;108(6):684–90.

54. Devereux RB, Dahlof B, Gerdts E, Boman K, Nieminen MS, Papademetriou V, et al. Regression of hypertensive left ventricular hypertrophy by losartan compared with atenolol: the Losartan Intervention for Endpoint Reduction in Hypertension (LIFE) trial. Circulation. 2004;110(11):1456–62.

55. Jondeau G, Boutouyrie P, Lacolley P, Laloux B, Dubourg O, Bourdarias JP, et al. Central pulse pressure is a major determinant of ascending aorta dilation in Marfan syndrome. Circulation. 1999;99(20):2677–81.

56. Milewicz DM, Guo DC, Tran-Fadulu V, Lafont AL, Papke CL, Inamoto S, et al. Genetic basis of thoracic aortic aneurysms and dissections: focus on smooth muscle cell contractile dysfunction. Annu Rev Genomics Hum Genet. 2008;9:283–302.

57. Ong KT, Perdu J, De Backer J, Bozec E, Collignon P, Emmerich J, et al. Effect of celiprolol on prevention of cardiovascular events in vascular Ehlers-Danlos syndrome: a prospective randomised, open, blinded-endpoints trial. Lancet. 2010;376(9751):1476–84.

58. Yetman AT, Bornemeier RA, McCrindle BW. Usefulness of enalapril versus propranolol or atenolol for prevention of aortic dilation in patients with the Marfan syndrome. Am J Cardiol. 2005;95(9):1125–7.

59. Riccioni G. Ivabradine: from molecular basis to clinical effectiveness. Adv Ther. 2010;27(3):160–7.

60. Fazel SS, Mallidi HR, Lee RS, Sheehan MP, Liang D, Fleischman D, et al. The aortopathy of bicuspid aortic valve disease has distinctive patterns and usually involves the transverse aortic arch. J Thorac Cardiovasc Surg. 2008;135(4):901–7, 7.e1–2.

61. Propanolol Aneurysm Trial Investigators. Propanolol for small abdominal aortic aneurysms: results of a randomized trial. J Vasc Surg. 2002;35(1):72–9.

62. Lindholt JS, Henneberg EW, Juul S, Fasting H. Impaired results of a randomised double blinded clinical trial of propranolol versus placebo on the expansion rate of small abdominal aortic aneurysms. Int Angiol. 1999;18(1):52–7.
63. Leach SD, Toole AL, Stern H, DeNatale RW, Tilson MD. Effect of beta-adrenergic blockade on the growth rate of abdominal aortic aneurysms. Arch Surg. 1988;123(5):606–9.
64. Hackam DG, Thiruchelvam D, Redelmeier DA. Angiotensin-converting enzyme inhibitors and aortic rupture: a population-based case–control study. Lancet. 2006;368(9536):659–65.
65. Sweeting MJ, Thompson SG, Brown LC, Greenhalgh RM, Powell JT. Use of angiotensin converting enzyme inhibitors is associated with increased growth rate of abdominal aortic aneurysms. J Vasc Surg. 2010;52(1):1–4.
66. Delbosc S, Alsac JM, Journe C, Louedec L, Castier Y, Bonnaure-Mallet M, et al. Porphyromonas gingivalis participates in pathogenesis of human abdominal aortic aneurysm by neutrophil activation. Proof of concept in rats. PLoS One. 2011;6(4):e18679.
67. Jackson V, Olsson T, Kurtovic S, Folkersen L, Paloschi V, Wagsater D, et al. Matrix metalloproteinase 14 and 19 expression is associated with thoracic aortic aneurysms. J Thorac Cardiovasc Surg. 2012;144(2):459–66.
68. Boyum J, Fellinger EK, Schmoker JD, Trombley L, McPartland K, Ittleman FP, et al. Matrix metalloproteinase activity in thoracic aortic aneurysms associated with bicuspid and tricuspid aortic valves. J Thorac Cardiovasc Surg. 2004;127(3):686–91.
69. Yang HH, Kim JM, Chum E, van Breemen C, Chung AW. Effectiveness of combination of losartan potassium and doxycycline versus single-drug treatments in the secondary prevention of thoracic aortic aneurysm in Marfan syndrome. J Thorac Cardiovasc Surg. 2010;140(2):305–12.e2.
70. Xiong W, Knispel RA, Dietz HC, Ramirez F, Baxter BT. Doxycycline delays aneurysm rupture in a mouse model of Marfan syndrome. J Vasc Surg. 2008;47(1):166–72; discussion 72.
71. Chung AW, Yang HH, Radomski MW, van Breemen C. Long-term doxycycline is more effective than atenolol to prevent thoracic aortic aneurysm in marfan syndrome through the inhibition of matrix metalloproteinase-2 and −9. Circ Res. 2008; 102(8):e73–85.
72. McLoughlin D, McGuinness J, Byrne J, Terzo E, Huuskonen V, McAllister H, et al. Pravastatin reduces Marfan aortic dilation. Circulation. 2011;124(11 Suppl):S168–73.

Chapter 4
Marfan Syndrome

**Gisela Teixido-Tura, Valentina Galuppo,
and Arturo Evangelista**

Abbreviations

ACEI	Angiotensin-converting enzyme inhibitors
Ang-II	Angiotensin-II
ARB	Angiotensin-II Receptor Blockers
AT1R	Angiotensin-II type 1 receptor
AT2R	Angiotensin-II type 2 receptor
BP	Blood pressure
CCB	Calcium-channel blockers
COX	cyclooxygenase
CT	Computed tomography
FBN1	Fibrillin-1
MFS	Marfan syndrome
MMP	Matrix metalloproteinase
MMPI	Matrix metalloproteinase inhibitor
MRI	Magnetic resonance imaging
PWV	Pulse wave velocity

G. Teixido-Tura, MD, PhD • V. Galuppo, MD
A. Evangelista, MD, FESC (✉)
Division of Cardiology, Hospital Universitari
Vall d'Hebron, Barcelona, Spain
e-mail: aevangel@vhebron.net

A. Evangelista, C.A. Nienaber (eds.), *Pharmacotherapy
in Aortic Disease*, Current Cardiovascular Therapy, Vol. 7,
DOI 10.1007/978-3-319-09555-4_4,
© Springer International Publishing Switzerland 2015

TAA   Thoracic aortic aneurysm
TGF-β Transforming growth factor-β
VSMC   Vascular smooth muscle cells

Introduction

Marfan syndrome (MFS) is a hereditary connective tissue disorder caused by mutations in FBN1. The gene encoding fibrillin-1 protein (FBN1) is located in chromosome 15 (position 15q21.1) and more than 1,000 different mutations have been described [1]. MFS has an autosomal dominant inheritance with high penetrance and high intra- and inter–familial variability, with an estimated prevalence of 1 case per 3,000–5,000 individuals. In approximately 75 % of cases, an individual inherits the disorder from an affected parent. The remaining 25 % result from a *de novo* mutation. Cardinal manifestations in MFS involve ocular, skeletal and cardiovascular systems. Ocular manifestations include ectopia lentis, myopia, retinal detachment and glaucoma. Skeletal involvement include scoliosis, bone overgrowth, joint laxity and chest deformities (pectus carinatum and excavatum). Cardiovascular manifestations include proximal ascending aorta dilatation, proximal main pulmonary artery dilatation and mitral valve prolapse. Aortic and/or mitral valve regurgitation related to structural primary abnormalities may be present.

Diagnosis

Despite the significant progress made in understanding the molecular and genetic basis of MFS, its diagnosis continues to depend primarily on clinical features that have been codified in the reviewed Ghent diagnostic nosology, described in 2010 [2], in which the coexistence of lens dislocation and aortic root aneurysm or dissection suffices to confirm the clinical diagnosis of MFS (Table 4.1). A family history of MFS and FBN1 mutation – known to be associated with

TABLE 4.1 Revised Ghent criteria for diagnosis of Marfan syndrome [2]

Absence of family history	Aortic root dilatation[a] or aortic root dissection AND ectopia lentis
	Aortic root dilatation[a] or aortic root dissection AND FBN1 mutation
	Aortic root dilatation[a] or aortic root dissection AND systemic score ≥ 7 points (see Table 4.2)
	Ectopia lentis AND FBN1 mutation that has been identified in an individual with aortic involvement
Presence of family history of Marfan syndrome	Aortic root dilatation[b] or aortic root dissection
	Ectopia lentis
	Systemic score ≥ 7 points

FBN1 fibrillin-1

[a]Aortic root Z-score ≥ 2. Z-score calculator can be found at http://www.marfan.org/dx/zscore

[b]Aortic root Z-score ≥ 2 above 20 years, ≥ 3 below 20 years

aortic manifestations – also contributes to the diagnosis. The remaining cardinal manifestations of Marfan syndrome are incorporated to a systemic score (Table 4.2). When this score is ≥ 7, it also contributes to the diagnosis. Therefore, a comprehensive multidisciplinary approach involving cardiac, orthopaedic, ophthalmological, and genetic consultations and testing are warranted to confirm the diagnosis.

Limitations of genetic testing include the following: (1) the mutation in the fibrillin-1 gene can cause conditions other than Marfan-like disorders; (2) none of the current methods used to find mutations in the fibrillin-1 gene identify all mutations that cause MFS; and (3) family members with the same mutation causing MFS may present a wide range of clinical manifestations.

TABLE 4.2 Systemic features in Marfan syndrome

System	Manifestation	Points for systemic score
Skeletal	Pectus carinatum	2 points
	Pectus excavatum	Or chest asymmetry: 1 point
	Scoliosis or spondylolisthesis	1 point
	Reduced upper to lower segment	When both are present without severe scoliosis. 1 point
	Increased arm-span to height ratio (dolicostenomelia)	
	Aracnodactilia	Wrist and thumb signs: both signs = 3 points; one sign = 1 point
	Hindfoot deformity	2 points
	Pes planus	1 point
	Protrusio acetabulae	2 points
	Reduced extension of the elbows (<170°)	1 point
	Facial appearance: dolicocephaly, malar hypoplasia, enophtalmos, retrognathia, down-slanting palpebral fissures	In the presence of 3 of the 5 = 1 point
	Highly arched palate with dental crowding	Not considered

(continued)

TABLE 4.2 (continued)

System	Manifestation	Points for systemic score
Ocular	Ectopia lentis	Major criteria
	Myopia	> 3 diopters = 1 point
	Retinal detachment	Not considered
	Glaucoma	Not considered
Cardiovascular	Aortic dilatation with or without aortic regurgitation	At the level of aortic root is a major criteria (see Table 4.1)
	Aortic dissection	Ascending aorta dissection is a major criteria (see Table 4.1)
	Mitral prolapse with or without mitral regurgitation	1 point
	Pulmonary artery dilatation	Not considered
	Mitral annulus calcification in individuals younger than 40 years	Not considered
Pulmonary	Spontaneous pneumothorax	2 points
	Apical blebs	Not considered
Integumentary	Stretch marks	1 point
	Recurrent or incisional herniae	Not considered
Dura	Lumbosacral dural ectasia	By CT or MR: 2 points

CT computed tomography, *MR* magnetic resonance

Complications

The main complication in patients with MFS is progressive aortic root enlargement, initially occurring at the sinuses of Valsalva. Ascending aortic aneurysm can precipitate acute type A aortic dissection or aortic rupture, and these complications were the primary cause of death before the advent of successful preventive therapies. Aortic aneurysm may develop early in children with MFS and the incidence rises during childhood and adolescence [3, 4]. Although early diagnosis has increased the median life span from around 40 to approximately 70 years, patients with MFS continue to suffer important morbidity [5]. Up to 90 % of Marfan patients will have cardiovascular events during their lifetime, including surgical repair of aortic root, aortic dissection or mitral valve surgery [6].

The current management of aortic involvement in MFS includes regular imaging follow-up to detect and quantify aortic dilation progression, and prophylactic aortic repair when aortic dilatation reaches a sufficient size sufficient to threaten dissection or cause aortic regurgitation. Prior to the era of open-heart surgery, the majority of patients with MFS died prematurely of aortic rupture, with an average life expectancy of 45 years [7]. The success of current medical and surgical treatment of aortic disease in MFS has substantially improved the average life expectancy, prolonging it up to 70 years [5, 8]. Thus, the major target for improving survival in patients with MFS is to prevent or delay aortic dissection.

Imaging Predictors of Complications

Several indices are associated with increased risk of a life-threatening aortic event. First among these is the absolute size of the proximal aorta [9, 10]. Aortic size ≥ 5.0 cm is strongly predictive of a high risk of aortic dissection and rupture [3], and surgical intervention at that stage is key. The "normal" diameter of the aorta is directly proportional to body size throughout normal growth and into adulthood.

Given their above average stature and therefore greater body surface area, growing individuals with MFS should have their aortic measurements indexed to body surface area [10]. This can be expressed as an aortic size ratio based on sex- and body size–related norms or expressed in relation to the normal aortic size distribution in the population as a Z score. When considered in these terms, patients with MFS with proximal aortic ratios ≥ 1.3 or Z scores ≥ 3 are at particular risk. However, Marfan syndrome has interesting nuances. For example, adiposity is often reduced in young patients; therefore, the body surface area calculated from standard formulae will underestimate the expected diameters of the proximal aorta and result in a higher Z score. Moreover, adults tend to accumulate central adiposity in adulthood, which will increase the calculated body surface area and reduce the apparent degree of aortic dilatation. Adults who gain weight after skeletal maturity will appear to have an improved aortic Z score. In such instances, focus on the absolute diameter and its changes is appropriate. In addition, the existing "aortic growth curves" are divided into children and young adults; interestingly, the curves do not overlap accurately. This poses problems for the clinician managing patients passing from adolescence to adulthood. Additionally, a common question is whether tall adults should have larger aortic diameters, even beyond those considered to be normal. Svensson et al. [11, 12] proposed an index (area of aortic root/ height >10 cm^2/m) to indicate surgery in patients with MFS. In addition to absolute aortic dimensions, the rate of change in size of the proximal aortic root over time is important. Even at relatively normal absolute aortic dimensions, a rapid increase in aortic size (>0.5 cm/year) portends an increased risk of dissection. However, to assume annual enlargement requires strict imaging quality control and re-measurement of aorta size at the same level and side by side. Additionally, a family history of early aortic complications is strongly predictive of decreased event-free survival [13]. Finally, diminished aortic compliance measured echocardiographically or by other means has been related to progressive aortic dilatation in

MFS patients [14, 15], although it is rarely measured on a routine clinical basis. Also of importance is the fact that patients with MFS can die from other cardiovascular complications, particularly severe mitral regurgitation (especially in children with a severe phenotype) and dysrhythmia [16].

Pathophysiology of Aortic Dilatation

The earliest recognition of the tissue abnormalities underlying aortic dilatation in MFS was medial layer degeneration, with fragmentation, disarray and loss of elastic lamina, and replacement by basophilic-staining proteoglycan. Electron microscopy in humans and in a mouse model of MFS demonstrated extracellular matrix disarray, with shrunken smooth muscle cell fibres, thickened basal membranes, abnormalities of collagen fibre structure and progressive fragmentation and loss of elastic lamellae [17]. The process is associated with signs of ongoing inflammation and matrix metalloproteinase activation [18, 19].

Fibrillin-1 is a major protein component of the microfibrils in the extracellular matrix and, as a result of its alteration, fragmentation and disarray of elastic fibres occur. However, not all manifestations of MFS (e.g. bone overgrowth) can be attributed to these structural abnormalities. In recent years, basic research has led to the notion that fibrillin-1 microfibrils also exert significant regulatory effect on cytokin-transforming growth factor-β (TGF-β) [20].

TGF-β molecules are cytokines synthesised and secreted by smooth muscle cells as inactive precursors in the form of a latent complex which is stored in the extracellular matrix [21, 22]. The fibrillins and latent TGF-β–binding proteins constitute a family of structurally-related proteins and participate in the sequestration of latent complexes of TGF-β and maintain them inactive. In the presence of deficient fibrillin-1, a lesser amount of TGF-β is inactivated and leads to an increase in TGF-β activity. Excessive TGF-β signalling – made evident by increased smad-2 phosphorylation – explains many of the manifestations found in Marfan syndrome: cystic lungs, mixomatous mitral valve leaflets and aortic dilatation [20, 23].

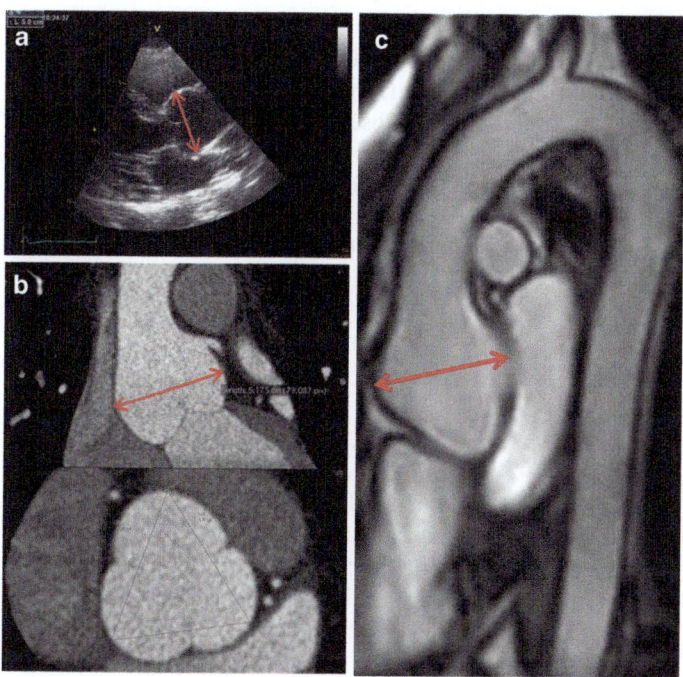

FIGURE 4.1 Imaging techniques for the study of the aorta in Marfan syndrome. (**a**) Transthoracic echocardiography; (**b**) computed tomography; (**c**) magnetic resonance imaging

Management

Although survival in these patients has improved dramatically in recent decades, mainly due to improved surgical techniques, most deaths in MFS patients are still due to aortic complications [5]. Routine aortic imaging by echo and/or MRI and CT is the recommended follow-up for these patients (Fig. 4.1), and elective aortic root surgery is considered when aortic root size is ≥50 mm [24]. However, medical treatment is needed to prevent aortic complications. As in other aortic conditions, strict blood pressure (BP) control is recommended. However, in MFS, medical treatment is considered to be prophylactic, even in the absence of high blood pressure, with the aim of reducing haemodynamic stress. The main aim of this chapter is to depict evidences, advantages and limitations of the current knowledge of the pharmacological treatment of this disease. To this end, several drugs will be discussed: β-blockers, angiotensin receptor blockers (ARB), angiotensin-converting enzyme inhibitors (ACEI) and calcium antagonists. More recent approaches such as statins, doxycycline, will also be reported.

Pharmacological Treatment in Marfan Syndrome

Mechanisms of Pharmacological Treatment

Medical treatment aims to reduce aortic haemodynamic stress: β-blockers, ARB, ACEI, calcium channel blocker (CCB), and/or to reduce TGF-β signalling: ARB. Recently, metalloproteinase inhibitors (MMPI) or anti-inflammatory drugs have been proposed.

Biomechanical and Haemodynamic Effects

Blood pressure and biomechanical properties of the aorta such as elasticity and compliance are determinant factors in aortic diameter enlargement in MFS [14, 15]. Different studies demonstrated that aortic stiffness is significantly greater in MFS patients compared with healthy volunteers, thereby suggesting more severe wall disease in MFS [25–29].

In clinical practice, arterial stiffness can be non-invasively estimated by three principal methods: (1) estimation of pulse wave velocity (PWV) by measurement of pulse transit time, (2) analysis of the arterial pressure wave contour (i.e. augmentation index, %), and (3) direct stiffness estimation using measurements of diameter or arterial luminal cross-sectional area change during the cardiac cycle and distending pressure measured at the site of diameter changes (i.e. distensibility and compliance). Carotid-to-femoral ('aortic') PWV is considered the gold standard [30] although PWV can also be measured at other levels.

β-blocker therapy reduces the exposure of weakened, histologically-abnormal aortic tissue to haemodynamic stressors by both inotropic and chronotropic negative effects, and thereby slows aortic dilatation progression. The use of β-adrenergic blockade to reduce haemodynamic stress in the proximal aorta in Marfan syndrome was first suggested in 1971, on the basis of findings in malignant hypertension that a reduction in the rate of increase in aortic pressure over time (dP/dt) was more effective at lowering the risk of aortic dissection than could be explained by a reduction of blood pressure alone [31]. Subsequent small studies of β-blockade effects in animal models with aortic disease and in uncontrolled studies of MFS had varying results [32]. β-blockers have proved to have little effect on central aortic pulse pressure in hypertensive patients [33], which is one of the main determinants of ascending aortic dilatation [34]. In 1989, Yin et al. [35] gave intravenous propranolol to Marfan subjects with dilated aortas during diagnostic cardiac catheterisation and found that it increased the magnitude of aortic wave reflection, reduced arterial compliance and did not reduce the maximum acceleration of blood into the ascending aorta. Other authors reported that β-blockade increases peripheral vascular resistance, which in turn may increase central aortic pressure and wall stress [36]. More recent studies also assessed the effect of β-blockers on aortic biomechanical properties: Groenink et al. [37] studied aortic properties by MRI and found a positive response of aortic distensibility and pulse wave velocity to the acute (2 weeks) treatment with metoprolol or atenolol; Rios et al. [36] found a heterogeneous response of aortic stiffness assessed by echocardiography to long-term treatment with atenolol. They defined a subgroup of patients in whom aortic distensibility improved after chronic β-blockade, with a more pronounced effect in Marfan patients with aortic root diameters below 40 mm. Furthermore, one study demonstrated that treatment with atenolol may not have an effect on the biomechanical properties of the aorta in paediatric patients with Marfan syndrome [38].

Recently, Nebivolol, a beta-1 receptor blocker with nitric oxide potentiating vasodilatory effects, has been proposed as a more appropriate choice than atenolol. In patients with hypertension, it reduces central pulse pressure and augmentation index more than atenolol, and it reduces central arterial pressure and left-ventricular hypertrophy more than metoprolol [39, 40].

Although one study assessed the role of aortic stiffness in predicting progressive aortic dilatation [14], the real clinical impact of the potential effect of β-blockade on aortic stiffness and aortic complications remains unclear.

Calcium-channel blockers reduce central aortic pressure in adult hypertensive patients [41], however similar effects have not been described in patients with MFS.

Angiotensin-converting enzyme inhibitors (ACEI) reduce angiotensin II (Ang-II) formation and are also known to reduce arterial stiffness in patients with different pathological conditions. More importantly, this ability seems to be independent of their ability to reduce BP. ACEI reduce central systolic pressure and conduit arterial stiffness, compared to β-blockers, in adults with hypertension [33].

One interesting study by Williams et al. [42] compared the haemodynamic and vascular effects of perindopril with those of two different drugs: atenolol and verapamil. Fourteen patients diagnosed of MFS were randomised (double-blinded) to receive 4 weeks of atenolol (75 mg), perindopril (4 mg) or verapamil (240 mg) in a cross-over design. Patients underwent a 2-week wash-out period prior to starting the protocol and after each treatment being switched to a new drug. Throughout the study, aortic diameter was assessed by transthoracic echocardiography, and arterial stiffness was measured as augmentation index and PWV (carotid-to-radial and carotid-to-femoral). Within-drug comparisons demonstrated that perindopril (-10.3 mmHg, $P = 0.002$), verapamil (-9.2 mmHg, $P = 0.003$) and atenolol (-7.1 mmHg, $P = 0.01$) reduced central systolic pressure and brachial pressure; central changes were the least and peripheral changes the greatest with atenolol; however between-drug comparisons were not significant. A trend was observed for augmentation to be reduced by perindopril (-6.3 %, $P = 0.05$), verapamil (-5.5 %, $P = 0.07$) and atenolol (-3.2 %, $P = 0.09$). The study results prove there were no statistically-significant differences among the drugs regarding aortic stiffness parameters. Only atenolol reduced heart rate (by 16 %) and delayed expansion in the arch and abdominal aorta (by 8 % and 11 %) ($P < 0.001$, $P < 0.01$ and $P < 0.05$, respectively, for inter-drug comparisons). Unexpectedly, atenolol did reduce central arterial pressure, although to a lesser degree than that observed with ACEI and CCB. This might be explained by a reduction in cardiac output (which fell by a mean of 17 %, $P = 0.24$) related to the reduction in heart rate (by a mean of 16 %, $P = 0.006$) rather than any change in stroke volume (12 %, $P = 0.22$). Alternatively, a negative inotropic effect would be expected to reduce the amplitude of aortic wave reflections during systole. This study suggested that a combination of a β-blocker with an ARB or an ACEI may be the most effective: while an ARB or ACEI may lower central pressures by reducing or delaying peripheral reflections, a β-blocker may reduce reflections by an effect on the left ventricle. This combination strategy is also being tested in some ongoing trials [43].

Molecular Effects

In order to reduce pathological molecular FBN1 mutation-derived mechanisms such as excessive TGF-β activation and signalling, different classes of drugs including ACEI and ARB have been investigated.

The creation of a mouse model of Marfan syndrome has significantly helped to further understanding of this disease. Overexpression of TGF-β explains many of the manifestations found in Marfan syndrome: cystic lungs, mixomatous mitral-valve leaflets and aortic dilatation have been associated with an increase in TGF-β signalling [20, 23]. Moreover, the administration of TGF-β antagonists (polyclonal TGF-β-neutralising antibody or losartan) in mice prevented the occurrence of Marfan features [44].

Inactive TGF-β is secreted by smooth muscle cells as a large latent complex. This latent complex is sequestered by the extracellular matrix and kept inactive. Deficient fibrillin-1 leads not only to histological abnormalities in the extracellular matrix microfibrils and connective tissue weakness, but also to a decrease in TGF-β sequestration leading to excessive TGF-β activation.

TGF-β can signal either through a canonical pathway involving the signal transduction proteins, Smads [45], or through several non-canonical, Smad-independent pathways (MAP-kinase pathway). In the Smad-related pathway, elevated TGF-β levels induce Smad2 activation that regulates transcription and induce the production of MMP proteins, a family of zinc endopeptidases responsible for degradation of the extracellular matrix in aortic aneurysms. The action of this class of proteins on aortic wall weakness in Marfan syndrome exponentially improves the risk of aortic aneurysm and rupture.

Ang–II is a potent vasoconstrictor acting directly on vascular smooth muscle cells and on the sympathetic nervous system; it also stimulates secretion of the hormone aldosterone, causing volume expansion through sodium retention. At molecular level, Ang-II can promote cell migration, proliferation and hypertrophy. Most of these effects are determined by Ang-II binding to its receptors: AT receptor 1 (AT1R) and AT receptor 2 (AT2R). Although angiotensin II (AngII) mediates the progression of aortic aneurysm, the relative contribution of its type 1 (AT1R) and type 2 (AT2R) receptors remains unknown. Ang-II promotes cell proliferation and fibrosis and suppresses apoptosis when binding to its AT1R, whereas binding to its AT2R has opposite effects, including antiproliferative and anti-inflammatory effects that are beneficial in aortic wall homeostasis. The effects of AT1R stimulation are mediated, at least in part, by TGF-β. The selective AT1 receptor blocker (ARB) losartan blocks AT1R and interferes with processes that are detrimental to tissue in mice with MFS (and by extension, humans) while not affecting signalling through AT2 that produces beneficial effects.

ACEI, on the other hand, reduce Ang-II levels and therefore signalling through both receptors. Although both drugs proved to attenuate canonical TGF-β signalling in the aorta, only losartan inhibited TGF-β-mediated activation of extracellular signal–regulated kinase by allowing continued signalling through AT2.

Angiotensin-converting enzyme inhibitors (ACEI) prevent the conversion of angiotensin-I to Ang-II, thus limiting signalling through both AT receptors. On balance, however, it seems possible that the benefit of AT1-receptor antagonism achieved with ACE inhibitors could outweigh the potential negative influence of AT2-receptor blockade. Thus, although the rationale for the use of ACEI in Marfan syndrome includes their significant effect on TGF-β levels and activity, they proved to be less effective than the ARB losartan in a mouse model of MFS [46].

Treatment of affected mice with losartan, prenatally and continuing until 10 months of age, resulted in the preservation of proximal aortic elastic fibre histology and overall aortic diameter comparable to that of wild-type mice [44]. In contrast, mice with the same mutation treated with propranolol had elastic lamella disruption and dilated aortic roots comparable to those of affected mice treated with placebo [44]. When losartan therapy was initiated at 2 months of age, comparable to adolescence in humans, the histological abnormalities and dilatation were reversed. Although propranolol therapy was associated with a reduction in aortic growth rate, this effect was significantly less than that seen with losartan [44]. The results of this mouse model of MFS suggest that treatment with angiotensin receptor blockers potentially targets both the underlying tissue disorder and reduces haemodynamic stressors.

Telmisartan has the strongest binding affinity to AT1R in comparison with other ARBs including losartan [47]. Concretely, the rank order of binding affinity to AT1R is telmisartan > olmesartan > candesartan > valsartan ≥ losartan. If losartan achieves its effect on MFS through AT1R blockade mediated via downstream TGF-β signalling inhibition, telmisartan would be expected to be the most effective ARB because of its strongest binding affinity to AT1R. Future studies should determine, however, whether telmisartan is more effective than losartan in Marfan syndrome patients [48].

Matrix Metalloproteinase Inhibitors (MMPI) and Anti-inflammatory Drugs

Multiple factors such as haploinsufficiency, FBN1 proteolysis, abnormal TGF-β signalling, increased MMP expression and changes in cell matrix interaction contribute to the complex pathogenesis of this disorder. Collagens, laminins and elastin have multiple motifs that are able to interact with cell-surface receptors on macrophages and other inflammatory cells. Evidence is accumulating in support of the notion that inflammation may also play an important role in the development of thoracic aortic aneurysm in MFS.

Statins

HMG-CoA reductase inhibitors (statins) are the most potent class of drugs used to inhibit cholesterol biosynthesis. In addition to being the mainstay of cholesterol-lowering therapy, some studies reported more beneficial cardiovascular effects unrelated to lipid reduction, the so-called pleiotropic effects [49]. Interestingly, statins exert anti-inflammatory and atherosclerotic plaque stabilisation effects by down-regulating matrix metalloproteinase (MMPs) expression [50]. Upregulation of MMP enzymes, particularly MMP-2 and MMP-9, is involved in MFS aortic wall degeneration and aneurysm formation [51].

Experimental research on a MFS animal model compared the effect of one of the statin family molecules, pravastatin, to losartan (angiotensin-2 antagonist). In that study, two Marfan genetically-modified mouse groups received, respectively, pravastatin 0.5 g/L and losartan 0.6 g/L for 6 weeks. Results from the different treated groups were compared with a third group of Marfan-modified untreated mice and a control group without pathological mutations. Echocardiogram analysis showed a significantly beneficial effect of pravastatin in attenuating aortic root dilatation in a MFS model ($p < 0.01$) compared to a Marfan untreated group. This outcome was analogous in the losartan group ($p < 0.01$). Moreover, immunohistochemical analysis of the mural architecture of the aortic wall demonstrated that pravastatin significantly reduced the degree of elastic fibres lost in the medial layer ($p = 0.01$). However, the losartan effect on elastin preserve was greater than that of statins ($p < 0.01$). In addition, haematoxylin and eosin staining showed the presence of foci of damage (island of damage) in the aortic wall of all MFS groups. Even if the number of foci was lower in treated animals, with no statistical difference between the medical groups, this finding may suggest that aortic injury was triggered in all groups and then reduced by drugs. Statins have been shown to have a potential role in MFS therapy and, therefore, this class of drugs should be investigated as a combination therapy in MFS patients.

Doxycycline

Doxycycline, a tetracycline-class antibiotic, is a non-specific inhibitor of MMPs [52] and suppresses aneurysm formation in animal models and human abdominal aortic aneurysm [53, 54]. In Marfan syndrome, Chung et al. [55] demonstrated that long-term treatment with doxycycline, through the inhibition of MMP-2 and −9, was more effective than atenolol in preventing TAA in a mouse model of Marfan syndrome by preserving elastic fibre integrity, normalising vasomotor function and suppressing TGF-β upregulation.

Indomethacin

The complex pathogenesis of MFS involves changes in TGF-β signalling, increased MMP expression and fragmentation of the extracellular matrix. A number of studies demonstrated raised macrophage and T-cell counts in the ascending aorta of human or mouse models of MFS; however, the efficacy of anti-inflammatory therapy in mouse MFS models has not been assessed to date. In a recent study, FBN1-underexpressing mgR/mgR Marfan mice were treated with oral indomethacin [56]. Treatment was begun at the age of three weeks and continued for 8 weeks, after which the aortas of wild type as well as treated and untreated mgR/mgR mice were compared. Indomethacin treatment led to a statistically-significant reduction in aortic elastin degeneration and macrophage infiltration, as well as lessening of MMP-2, MMP-9 and MMP-12 upregulation. Additionally, indomethacin reduced both cyclooxygenase-2 (COX-2) expression and activity in the aorta of mgR/mgR mice. COX-2-mediated inflammatory infiltrate contributed to aortic aneurysm progression in mgR/mgR mice, providing evidence that COX-2 is a relevant therapeutic target in MFS associated aortic aneurysmal disease. Therefore, COX-2-mediated inflammatory infiltration plays an important role in the pathogenesis of aortic aneurysm disease in MFS. In another paper, the same team demonstrated that the non-steroidal anti-inflammatory drug indomethacin significantly improved elastin integrity and reduced the number of macrophages in the aortic adventitia of mgR/mgR mice, which coincided with decreased MMP-2, MMP-9 and MMP-12 expression. Based on these studies, the authors speculated that the macrophage infiltration observed in the aortic wall of mgR/mgR Marfan mice participates in a kind of vicious cycle, in which matrix fragments induce deleterious effects, including upregulation of MMP activity and macrophage infiltration, which in turn reinforces the pathological processes associated with matrix degradation and defects in TGF-β sequestration [57–59].

Medical Treatment Studies

Beta-Blockers

Beta-blockers are the standard medical treatment for the prevention of aortic dilatation in Marfan syndrome. Their positive benefit relies on their haemodynamic effects: reduction in the force of left ventricular ejection by negative inotropic and chronotropic effects leading to decreased aortic wall stress. Several studies reported that β-blockers delay aortic root dilatation (Table 4.3). However, those studies had major limitations: the majority were retrospective [5, 60–63] and others prospective but not randomised [64, 65]. The majority showed retardation of aortic root dilatation [62, 66–69], although two studies did not demonstrate this benefit [61, 70]. None of those studies convincingly demonstrated a benefit in overall morbidity and mortality. The strongest evidence comes from a prospective randomised open-label trial by Shores et al. [66] that included 70 patients with Marfan syndrome divided into a control group of 38 patients who received no treatment and a treatment group of 32 patients who received propranolol. Aortic follow-up was performed by echocardiography and aortic dilatation was evaluated with the slope of the regression line for aortic ratio evolution over time. In that study, propranolol slowed the rate of aortic dilatation compared to the control group. The authors defined *aortic ratio* as the ratio of the measured aortic diameter to the expected diameter and the slope of the regression line for the increase in aortic ratios over time. The slope for aortic ratio of the control group was 0.084 per year, whereas in the treatment group was only 0.023 per year ($p < 0.001$). Five patients in the treatment group, two of whom did not follow the propranolol regimen, and nine patients in the control group reached a composite clinical end-point, which was defined as heart failure, aortic dissection, cardiovascular surgery or death. That study supported the use of β-blockers, concretely propranolol, in patients with Marfan syndrome based on two findings: first, aortic dilatation was faster in patients in the control group than in the treatment group and second, more patients in the control group reached the composite clinical end-point than in the treatment group. The construction of a composite end-point was necessary since no single clinical end-point reached statistical significance on its own merit. Although the results were certainly promising, the authors concede that the study was neither placebo-controlled nor blind, with each patient and investigator aware of the

TABLE 4.3 Studies on β-blockers in Marfan syndrome

Author	Design	Treatment groups	Age (years)	Mean aortic root at baseline	Includes children	Includes operated patients	Follow-up	Aortic dilatation end-points	Results
Roman (1993)	Prospective observational Designed to assess the impact of aortic dilatation (no dilatation, localized to aortic root or generalized) and the presence of aortic complications	G1: β-blocker, not specified, N = 79 G2: None, N = 34	28 ± 15 yrs Range = 6 months – 66 yrs		Yes (n = 29)	No	49 ± 24 months		Similar number of complication (AD, AAS, ARP) between groups

| Shores (1994) | Randomised clinical trial Open-label | G1: Propranolol, N=32 G2: None, N=38 | G1: 15.4 yrs G2: 14.5 yrs | G1: 34.6 mm G2: 30.2 mm Significantly different | Excluded <12 yrs | No | G1=10.7 yrs G2=9.3 yrs | Aortic root by echo (M-mode) Slope of the regression line for aortic ratio over time | Lower aortic dilatation by echo (M-mode) over time in treatment group ($p<0.001$) Composite end-point (D, AD, AAS, CHF): 5 (15.6 %) in G1 and 9 in G2 (23.7 %). No statistical comparison reported |

(continued)

TABLE 4.3 (continued)

Author	Design	Treatment groups	Age (years)	Mean aortic root at baseline	Includes children	Includes operated patients	Follow-up	Aortic dilatation end-points	Results
Salim (1994)	Retrospective	G1 (Centre A or B): propranolol, atenolol, N=100 G2: None, N=13	G1: Centre A: 10.4±3.4 yrs Centre B: 14.1±3.4 yrs G2: 0.2±4.6 yrs	G1: Centre A: 31.1±7.0 mm Centre B 34.0±5.4 mm G2: 31.3± 7.4 mm P=NS	Yes	No	G1: Centre A: 5.5±2.7 yrs Centre B: 4.2±2.1 yrs G2: 5.7±1.8 yrs	Aortic root dilatation rate by echo (M-mode) in mm/year	Aortic ratios (mm/year): Centre A 1.1±1.1; Centre B 0.7±1.8; Control 2.1±1.6 (p<0.006 between centre A and control: p<0.003 between centre B and control)
Silverman (1995)	Retrospective This study was designed to describe Marfan life expectancy compared to a historical cohort	G1: Atenolol, Nadolol, Propranolol, Metoprolol, N=191 G2: None: N=226	G1: 33±14 yrs G2: 31±17 yrs		Yes	Yes	5.2±3.6 yrs	None	Median cumulative probability of survival 2 years longer in G1 (p=0.01)

Study	Design	Groups	Age	Baseline aortic dimensions			Follow-up	Method	Results
Legget (1996)	Retrospective Designed to examine the clinical and echocardiographic predictors of outcome in a cohort of patients with Marfan's syndrome	G1: β-blocker, not specified, for >12 months, N=30 G2: None, N=53	21±13 yrs Range 1-54 yrs		Yes	No	4 yrs	Aortic ratios, by bidimensional echo	No differences in aortic root growth No differences in actuarial freedom from all events (D, AAS, AD)
Rossi-Foulkes (1999)	Prospective Non-randomized Open-label	G1: β-blockers, N=20 G2: CCB, N=6 G3: None, N=27	9.4±5.3 yrs	G1+G2: 33±7 mm G3: 26±7 mm P<0.01 No differences in aortic diameters indexed by BSA	Yes, exclusively	No	44±24 months	Aortic root dimensions by bidimensional echo (absolute values and aortic ratios)	Medicated patients had slower aortic growth than the unmedicated patients (both absolute aortic growth rate 1.0±0.8 vs. 1.7±1.0, p < 0.05)

(continued)

Table 4.3 (continued)

Author	Design	Treatment groups	Age (years)	Mean aortic root at baseline	Includes children	Includes operated patients	Follow-up	Aortic dilatation end-points	Results
Selamet (2007)	Retrospective	G1: 27 atenolol, 1 propranolol and 1 metoprolol, N=29; G2: None, N=34	G1: 9.2±4.0 yrs; G2: 8.8±4.8 yrs	G1: 29.3±4.2 mm; G2: 29.7±7 mm; P=0.75	Yes, exclusively <18 yrs	No	G1: 76.3±31.0 months; G2: 81.3±53.9 months	Aortic root dimensions by bidimensional echo (absolute values and z-scores)	No differences in aortic root growth. Similar number of patients in each group achieved a clinical end-point (AAS, AD, D)

| Ladouceur (2007) | Retrospective | G1: Atenolol (70 %), nadolol (17 %) and propranolol (6 %), N=77, G2: None, N=78 | G1: 6.1 ±3.2 yrs G2 7.4 ±5.2 yrs | G1: 28.4 ± 4.8 mm G2: 27.2 ± 5.7 mm P=NS | Yes, exclusively <12 yrs | No | 4.5 ±3.7 yrs | Aortic root dimensions by bidimensional echo | Aortic root dilatation 1.05 mm/year in G1 compared to 1.15 mm/year in G2, p=0.0001 A trend toward lower cardiac mortality, decreased need for preventive aortic surgery, and less dissection was observed |

G1, G2, G3 groups of treatment, *yrs* years, *AD* aortic dissection, *AAS* ascending aorta surgery, *ARP* aortic regurgitation progression, *echo* echocardiography, *D* death, *CHF* cardiac heart failure, *NS* not significant, *CCB* calcium-channel blockers, *BSA* body surface area patient's group. Thus, although the results did show potential for β-blockers in Marfan patients, it is highly possible that the study's results were subject to bias and a placebo effect. Furthermore, although heart failure, dissection and death are hard end-points, the decision for surgery is a softer call and might have influenced the results.

Further, the study did not have a definitive means of ensuring patient compliance; patients in the treatment group may not have followed the correct propranolol dosage, and those in the control group may have taken other medications. The major limitation of the study, however, was the small sample size. By the end of the trial, the already minimal population had decreased by 20 % owing to clinical end-points. Although the authors appropriately believed the presence of more end-points in the control group supported their conclusions, a mere four-person difference between the control and treatment groups seems unconvincing, even more so when one takes into account that two of the deaths in the control group were unrelated to aortic complications. One year later, Silverman et al. [5] published a retrospective observational study in 417 Marfan patients treated at four different Marfan clinics. Although this study was thought to describe Marfan life expectancy compared to a historical cohort [7], the authors also reported that the 191 Marfan patients treated with β-blockers (atenolol, metroprolol, nadolol or propranolol) had a median cumulative probability of survival 2 years longer than those who had never taken β-blockers, 72 vs 70 years ($P<0.01$). However, the authors themselves admitted that the design of the study precluded the assessment of the contribution of β-blockers to increased survival. Roman et al. [9] published a prospective observational study designed to assess the prognostic significance of the type of aortic dilatation (localised to aortic root or generalised to aortic root and tubular ascending aorta) and found a similar number of aortic complications between patients with or without medical treatment (mainly β-blockers but also with other blood pressure lowering medications), 33 % vs 30 %. However, that study is difficult to analyse since it was not specifically designed to address β-blocker treatment in patients with Marfan syndrome. A paper published by Salim et al. [62] retrospectively studied 100 patients who received β-blockers (either propranolol or atenolol) at two specialised centres and compared them with a control group of 13 patients who refused treatment. The study found that patients in the treatment group had an aortic root growth rate of 1.1 mm per year, whereas patients in the control group had an aortic root growth rate of 2.1 mm per year (P < 0.006). The limited number of patients in the control group compared with the treatment group, however, renders it difficult to lend credence to the comparison. In 1996, Legget et al. [61] published another observational prospective study with the aim of defining a lower risk group for aortic complications depending on echocardiographic follow-up. In that study, 30 patients receiving β-blockers for least 1 year were compared with 80 patients who had not received β-blockers (or for less than 1 year) and found no differences in aortic root growth or aortic complications (death, need for surgery or aortic dissection).

Of the five previously-mentioned studies, only one [66] was a randomised clinical trial, three were not designed to study β-blocker effect on clinical outcome or aortic root growth [5, 9, 61] and one was a non-randomised prospective observational study [62].

A recent meta-analysis that included the five previous studies [5, 9, 61, 62, 66, 69] on β-blockers in Marfan concluded that there is no evidence that β-blockers have clinical benefit in patients with Marfan syndrome [71]. The above-mentioned studies mainly include young patients, so the effect of β-blockade in older ages is even less clear. On the other hand, two recent retrospective observational studies in children reported conflicting results: the first, published by Selamet et al. [63] retrospectively identified 63 Marfan patients (34 untreated and 29 treated with β-blockers) with echocardiographic follow-up and found no differences in the rates of change in aortic root measurements or aortic complications, with a mean follow-up of 81.3 vs 76.3 months in the untreated and treated groups, respectively. The second retrospective study by Ladouceur et al. [60] included 155 children (<12 years) with MFS and compared the 77 that received β-blockers to the 78 that had never received β-blockers; they reported a lower aortic dilatation rate and a trend towards a lower cardiac event rate (mean follow-up: 4.5 ± 3.7 years) in the patients treated with β-blockers.

The role of β-blockers in certain subsets of Marfan patients is even less clear. That is the case for the subgroup of non-dilated patients or those previously operated on.

Therefore, although β-blockade is the accepted and conventional treatment for MFS, and recommended by the American and European clinical guidelines [25, 72], the evidence for these recommendations is still weak and thus prospective, multicentre clinical trials are needed to assess the real efficacy of this therapy. Moreover, while receiving treatment with β-blockers, these patients eventually present aortic dilatation or dissection; consequently, more research is required to prevent aortic complications with medical treatment.

Calcium-Channel Blockers (CCB)

Calcium-channel blockers (CCB) are sometimes prescribed for patients with Marfan syndrome when β-blockers are contraindicated, for example in asthma; however, their use has been evaluated in only one small study: Rossi-Foulkes et al. [65] reported a slower rate of aorta enlargement in 26 patients receiving treatment, compared with placebo (+0.9 vs 1.8 mm/year, $p = 0.02$), but 20 of these patients received β-blockers and only six a calcium-channel blocker (including verapamil in five). No comparisons between the drugs were reported because the numbers were too small. Since verapamil is negatively inotropic and chronotropic and also causes generalised arterial and arteriolar dilatation, there are theoretical grounds for expecting benefit in Marfan syndrome; however, the drug has not been tested adequately. Calcium antagonists reduce central arterial pressure and stiffness [41]. A dihydropyridine calcium antagonist such as nifedipine or amlodipine might have similar effects on conduit arterial function, but might be less useful owing to the relative lack of effects on the cardiac inotropic state. However, at the American Heart Association Meeting in 2012 data were presented showing CCBs exacerbated aortic disease and caused premature lethality in MFS mice due to increased ERK activation [73]. Therefore, CCBs have to be used with caution in patients with MFS.

Angiotensin-Converting Enzyme Inhibitors

Angiotensin-converting enzyme inhibitors (ACEI) are used either alone or in combination with β-adrenoceptor blockers. The pharmacological rationale is the involvement of the renin-angiotensin system in the development of aortic stiffening, dilatation and rupture in Marfan syndrome (Fig. 4.2).

ACEI reduce central arterial pressure and conduit arterial stiffness [41]. Preliminary evidence suggests that they may be useful in Marfan syndrome. In hypertension studies, it has been suggested that perindopril may reduce large arterial stiffness by a mechanism that is independent of its direct effect on lowering blood pressure [74]. ACEI have other effects that might also be clinically useful in patients with Marfan syndrome. Activation of the Ang-II AT2 plays an important role in promoting apoptosis of VSMCs and cystic medial degeneration in Marfan syndrome [75]. A study by Nagashima et al. [76] demonstrated that an ACEI (but not an Ang-II AT1R blocker) prevented cystic medial degeneration, apoptosis of VSMCs, and aortic dissection in rats.

Different authors hypothesised that ACE inhibitors may be a useful treatment for reducing aortic dilatation in MFS patients. The first randomised, double-blind, placebo-controlled trial of ACE inhibitors in MFS patients was conducted in 2007 [77]. In that study, 10 MFS patients with normal end-diastolic aortic diameter were randomly assigned to perindopril and compared with 7 similar MFS control patients. At baseline, echocardiographic variables were similar between the two groups. Perindopril dose was raised from

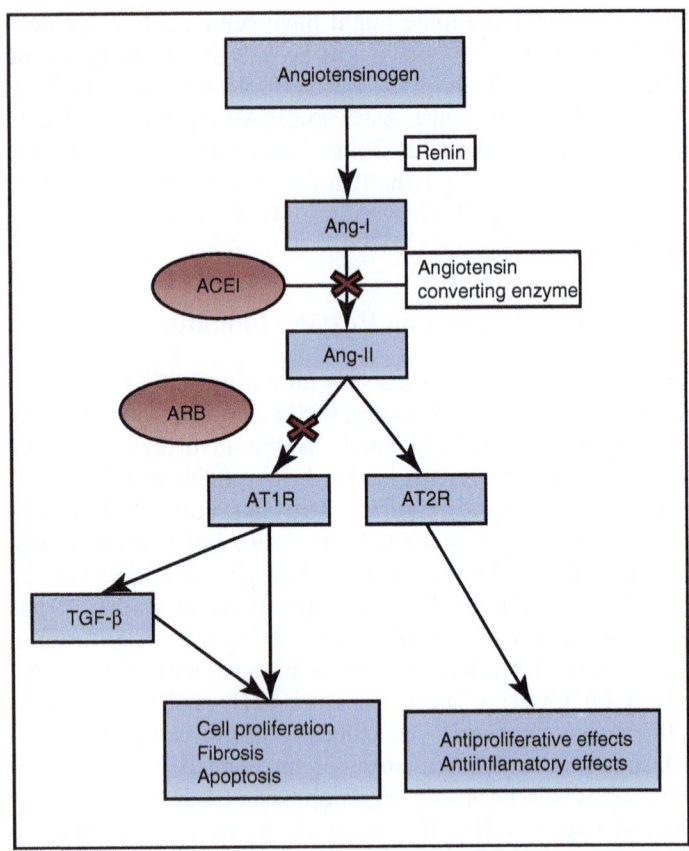

FIGURE 4.2 Renin-angiotensin system in the aorta and sites for drug treatment. *Ang-I* angiotensin-I, *Ang-II* angiotensin-II, *ACEI* angiotensin-converting enzyme inhibitors, *ARB* angiotensin-II receptor blockers, *AT1R* angiotensin-II receptor type 1, *AT2R* angiotensin-II receptor type 2, *TGF-β* transforming growth factor-β

2 to 8 mg/day over the first 3 weeks of the 24-week study. Importantly, both groups of patients were receiving long-term treatment with a β-blocker. During the study, indices of arterial stiffness were assessed by carotid tonometry, Doppler velocimetry, and pulse-wave velocity (PWV) readings.

Covariate analysis proved that perindopril significantly reduced central and peripheral PWV ($p < 0.001$) and carotid pulse pressure ($p = 0.03$), compared with controls. These changes in aortic stiffness parameters in perindopril group remained significant even when mean arterial pressure was included as a covariate. The main result of this study was that perindopril reduced the aortic growth rate compared to controls over a 24-week period. Aortic size was followed by two-dimensional and M-mode echocardiography. The end-diastolic aortic root diameter was significantly reduced in the perindopril group (1.2–3.0 mm/m^2) compared to the control group. Improvements in arterial stiffness and aortic diameter were independent of arterial pressure. In addition, biochemical analysis showed that perindopril reduced Ang-II production and signalling via both AT1R and AT2R-dependent pathways. Owing to the inhibition of AT1R signalling, ACE inhibitor-treated patients showed significantly reduced levels of the TGF-β cytokine ($p < 0.02$) and its downstream messengers, with levels of MMP-2 and MMP-3 dropping ($p < 0.001$ for both) compared with placebo at 24 weeks.

Interestingly, Williams et al. [42] reported a small but significant reduction (6 %) of the sinotubular junction aortic diameter after 4 weeks of perindopril treatment ($p = 0.024$). No differences were observed at sinuses de Valsalva level.

Despite the potential usefulness of ACEI, these studies are limited because of their small sample size and short duration, therefore the results remain weak and confounding.

A recent non-randomised trial compared enalapril to either atenolol or propranolol (propranolol was given to children <12.5 kg) in 57 subjects, mean age 14.6 and 12 years, respectively [64], in the ACEI and β-blocker groups. Mean follow-up was 3.0 ± 0.2 years. Increased aortic distensibility (3.0 ± 0.3 vs 1.9 ± 0.4 cm^2/dyn; $p < 0.02$) and reduced aortic stiffness index (8.0 ± 2.9 vs 18.4 ± 3.8; $p < 0.05$) were seen in the enalapril group compared with the β-blocker group and this resulted in a smaller increase in aortic root diameter (0.1 ± 1.0 vs 5.8 ± 5.2 mm; $p < 0.001$). Nine subjects underwent aortic root replacement during the study, two in the enalapril group

(6 %) and seven while receiving β-blockers (28 %). Marfan patients treated with ACEI had a reduced aortic growth rate and a lower event rate compared with those treated with β-blockers. However, as that study was non-randomised, treating physicians had a choice of β-blocker or enalapril, leading to a potential for confounding by indication, and the doses of drugs were not optimised by any consistent criteria. Patients with perceived lower risk could have preferentially been treated with enalapril, whereas high-risk patients would more likely have been steered toward β-blockade as "standard of care." The presence of significantly lower aortic distensibility and a higher stiffness index in the β-blocker group suggests that such a differential therapy choice did exist. The authors gave three possible mechanisms for the beneficial effect of the ACE inhibitor: the first was inhibition of VSMC apoptosis as described above; the second was a bradykinin-mediated improvement in aortic elastic tone; and the third was blocking of hyperhomocysteinaemia which increases vascular stiffness and reduction in MMP activity [78].

Angiotensin-II Receptor Blockers (ARB)

Losartan, an Ang-II AT1R antagonist, has been the object of major investigations. Losartan not only lowers blood pressure — a desirable effect in patients with aortic conditions — but has also previously demonstrated antagonism of TGF-β in animal models in different conditions [79, 80]. After the publication of results from a mouse model of MFS, a first retrospective study on the effect of ARB in children with MFS was published by the group of Dietz et al. in 2008 [81]. In that study, 18 paediatric patients (14 months to 16 years of age) were identified as having received ARB (losartan in 17 and irbesartan in 1) after other medical therapy (β-blockers with or without ACEI) had failed to prevent aortic root enlargement. ARB was added to their previous medical treatment and patients were receiving the maximal weight-based dose within 6 months after the initiation of therapy (losartan target dose was 1.4 mg/kg of body weight per day and irbesartan 2.0 mg per kilogram of body weight per day) and received the treatment for at least 1 year. If previous treatment was ACEI, it was discontinued. With clinical and echocardiographic follow-up between 12 and 47 months, a significant reduction was demonstrated in the progression of aortic root enlargement: change in aortic root diameter decreased significantly from 3.54 ± 2.87 mm/year during the previous medical therapy to 0.46 ± 0.62 mm/year during ARB therapy ($p < 0.001$). Moreover, a statistically-significant reduction was also observed at sinotubular junction level ($p < 0.05$). The authors simultaneously identified a group of 65 Marfan paediatric patients with milder aortic root disease (aortic root diameter z-score 3.25 ± 1.52 vs. 6.52 ± 2.43 in the ARB group, $p < 0.001$) that only received β-blockers during follow-up. Mean rates of change in aortic root diameter (1.71 ± 1.24 mm per year) and in aortic root diameter z-score (0.24 ± 0.50 per year) in the patients that received β-blockers alone were significantly higher than those in severely affected patients receiving ARB therapy ($P < 0.001$ for both comparisons). However, that study had several limitations: (1) small population sample; (2) non-randomised, retrospective and observational study; (3) all patients had severe aortic root enlargement or a rapid increase in aortic diameters before ARB therapy started. However, the results were very encouraging and led to the design of many clinical trials — the majority are still ongoing — to assess the efficacy of ARB versus β-blockers, added to β-blockers, compared to no additional treatment or to placebo in Marfan patients.

The first clinical trial on ARB in Marfan syndrome was published in 2013 by Groenink et al. (COMPARE trial) [82]. This was a randomised, multicentre (four centres), open-label clinical trial with blinded assessment of end-points that included 233 Marfan patients over the age of 18 years (38 ± 13 years, 47 % females) with no history of previous aortic dissection or aortic root diameter >50 mm. Patients were randomised to receive either losartan ($n = 116$) or no additional treatment ($n = 117$) added to their previous medical treatment. Patients in the losartan group were started on

50 mg daily and this dose was doubled after 2 weeks. Maximum losartan dosage of 100 mg daily was achieved in 54 % of patients. Previous medical treatment was β-blockers in 70.1 % of the control group and 75 % of the losartan and CCB group in 2.6 and 1.7 % respectively. Mean follow-up was 3.1 ± 0.4 years.

The primary end-point was the aortic dilatation rate assessed by magnetic resonance imaging (MRI) at six pre-defined aortic levels from the aortic root to bifurcation. The aortic root could be evaluated in 145 patients with a native aortic root. Baseline aortic root diameters were similar between both treatment groups (43.8 ± 5.0 vs. 43.2 ± 4.4 mm, $P = 0.436$). The aortic root dilatation rate was significantly lower in the losartan group than in the control group, 0.77 ± 1.36 vs. 1.35 ± 1.55 mm/3 years, respectively, $P = 0.014$. The percentage of participants with a stable aortic root (defined as a dilatation rate ≤0 mm/3 years) was 50 % in the losartan group and 31 % in the control group ($P = 0.022$). The aortic dilatation rate beyond the aortic root was evaluated in 218 patients and was not significantly reduced by losartan. This study included 63 patients with previous aortic root replacement (27 in the losartan group). As expected, baseline aortic dimensions in the remaining aortic trajectory were greater in this previously operated group when compared with the total patient cohort. Although in this subgroup of patients, the aortic arch dilatation rate was significantly lower in the losartan group than in the control group (0.50 ± 1.26 vs. 1.01 ± 1.31 mm/3 years, respectively, $P = 0.033$), patients ran-domised to losartan demonstrated smaller dimensions at baseline of the aortic arch and the descending thoracic aorta at the level of the diaphragm compared with the control group (respectively, 24 ± 3 vs. 26 ± 4 mm, $P = 0.029$ and 21 ± 2 vs. 23 ± 4 mm, $P = 0.009$).

Moreover, in the overall cohort, no differences in separate clinical end-points or the composite end-point were found between groups (prophylactic aortic root surgery: 10 vs. 8, distal aortic surgical intervention: 0 vs. 1, type B aortic dissection: 0 vs. 2, for the losartan and control groups, respectively). No cardiovascular deaths occurred during the study. Study limitations include the open-label design of the trial.

A non-randomised interventional study with no control group was published by Pees et al. [83] in 2013; this study included 20 children and young adults (mean age 11.3 ± 6.3 years) with genetically-confirmed MFS that initiated treatment with losartan. Ten of the 20 patients received losartan monotherapy as their first medication, 8 stopped their previous treatment with β-blockers and initiated losartan and 2 received losartan plus a β-blocker. Aortic follow-up (33 ± 11 months) was performed by echocardiography and showed a significant reduction in the normalised aortic dimensions at the level of the aortic root (-3.0 ± 2.8 mm/m^2, $p < 0.001$), sino-tubular junction (-1.5 ± 2.3 mm/m^2, $p = 0.012$), and ascending tubular aorta (-2.1 ± 2.0 mm/m^2, $p = 0.001$). This last study had several major issues: (1) lack of a control group; (2) the results expressed as a reduction in indexed aortic diameters by body surface area when, in this age period, body growth may predominate over aortic growth, thereby explaining the results.

Another observational study by Mueller et al. was published in 2014 [84]. In that study, a cohort of 215 patients (mean age 9.01 ± 5.7 years) was retrospectively identified and 40 untreated and unoperated patients were selected. Clinical and echocardiographic follow-up was performed after ARB and/or β-blockers were initiated. Twenty-two patients received ARB therapy and 18 received β-blockers. Mean follow-up in the β-blocker group was 5.51 ± 3.30 years vs 1.4 ± 0.24 years in the ARB group ($p < 0.001$). Both medications showed a significant and similar reduction in sinus of Valsalva dilatation (evaluated as z-score). However, this study lacked of a control group, so it is not clear what the natural evolution of the z-score was in an untreated group of this age.

In 2013, Chiu et al. [85] published a clinical trial on a paediatric population to confirm the superiority of combined therapy with β-blockers and ARB vs the use of β-blockers alone in Marfan patients. In that study, 28 patients (aged 13.1 ± 6.3 years) with aortic root dilatation (z-score >2) were randomised to receive β-blockers (atenolol or propanolol) or β-blockers and ARB (losartan). In the monotherapy β-blocker group, the maximum dose of atenolol or propanolol was 150 mg/day for adults and 2 mg/kg per day for children. In the combined therapy group, the adult target dosage of losartan was 100 mg/day (or the maximum tolerable dose) and the paediatric dose was started at 0.7 mg/kg/day and increased gradually up to 50 mg/day. Moreover, in the latter group, β-blocker doses were reduced (atenolol 50 mg/day, propanolol 20 mg/bid) to decrease pharmacologic cross-interactions. Patients with a history of aortic surgery or severe aortic disease (aortic root diameter at sinus of Valsalva level >55 mm, or aortic diameter growth >1 mm/year) were excluded. The follow-up trial lasted 3 years. The aortic diameter of patients was checked every 3–4 months by transthoracic echocardiography. Emphatically, the results showed that combined therapy (β-blocker + losartan) reduced the annual dilatation rate of aortic root compared to β-blocker therapy alone (respectively 0.10 mm/year vs 0.89 mm/year, respectively; p = 0.02). Moreover, the study found a significant reduction in aortic diameter relative to baseline in 33 % of patients in the combined group but in none of those receiving β-blockers alone. Importantly, changes in aortic diameters were significantly less in the combined group at all ascending aorta levels (sinus of Valsalva, p = 0.02; aortic root z score, p = 0.04; aortic annulus, p = 0.03; and sinotubular junction, p = 0.03). However, no significant changes in blood pressure after medication use occurred in either group. Moreover, no changes were found either in descending aorta, aortic stiffness, and cross-sectional compliance. Even if that study was limited to a small population, it showed the potential benefit of ARB drugs added to standard therapy in Marfan patients.

Regarding losartan treatment, it is important to bear in mind that impressive results obtained in mice cannot be directly extrapolated to general medical therapy in MFS patients. It should be emphasised that, in animal models, losartan was administered in the first months of life or during pregnancy in the embryogenesis phase.

Ongoing Clinical Trials

The pharmacological prophylactic management of MFS has moved somewhat beyond the Marfan mouse stage to humans, although considerable insights are still being gained from such animal studies. With the use of losartan, an AT1R inhibitor licensed for other conditions, the translational path has been considerably shortened. The next crucial event is publication of the results of the ongoing randomised controlled trials. An increasing problem in the testing of novel hypotheses generated by new molecular insights into Marfan syndrome is that the small patient population can only sustain a limited number of trials. In this respect, there is no strong evidence to suggest that any of the AT1R antagonists are any better than losartan.

Ongoing trials are listed on the clinical trial homepage http://www.clinicaltrials.gov, see also Table 4.4.

The *USA trial* is comparing β-blocker therapy (atenolol) directly with losartan in an open-label, randomised trial [86]. The study will eventually include 600 patients with an age range of 0.5–20 years and a follow-up period by echo of 3 years. This study evaluates the advantages of two different first-line therapies but not the benefit of combining the two drugs compared with up-to-date standard therapy.

The *French MARFANSARTAN trial* [87] is a multicentre randomised placebo-controlled trial evaluating the efficacy of losartan in limiting aortic dilatation in MFS patients aged 10 years or older receiving standard therapy (β-blocker or calcium channel blocker if β-blocker therapy is not tolerated). Patients who had previously undergone aortic surgery were excluded. Aortic root diameter will be measured using two-dimensional echocardiography in a 3-year follow-up period. The desired number of patients included will be 300.

The *Italian trial* (**MaNeLo**) [43] is comparing three different approaches: β-blocker or losartan alone or the combination of both. The β-blocker being used (nebivolol) carries theoretical advantages over the non-selective propanolol used in the landmark study of Shores et al. [66] and over the

TABLE 4.4 Ongoing clinical trials on ARB in Marfan syndrome

First author (country)	Name and identification number	Study design and objectives	Year trial started – estimated completion	Follow-up	Estimated enrolment	Age	Aortic size at entry	Drug and daily dosage	Control drug and daily dosage
Lacro et al. (USA)	NCT 00429364	Randomized, SB Losartan vs Atenolol	Jan 2007– Feb 2014	3 years	604	6 months to 25 years	Z-score >3	Losartan 0.3– 1.4 mg/kg	Atenolol 0.5–4 mg/kg
Delaint et al. (France)	MARFANSARTAN trial NCT 00763893	Randomized, DB Losartan vs placebo (+ standard therapy: propranolol)	Sep 2008– Mar 2014	3 years	303	>10 years	ND	Losartan 50 mg/day if <50 kg; 100 mg/day if >50 kg	Placebo
Gambarin et al. (Italy)	MaNeLo trial NCT 00683124	Randomized, DB Losartan vs Nebivolol or combination of both	July 2008– July 2013	4 years	291	1–55 years	Z-score ≥2; or absolute aortic root diameter >38 mm for females and >40 mm for males	Losartan 100 mg/day for adults and 1.5 mg/kg/d for children <16 years	Nebivolol alone or combined 10 mg/ day for adults and 0.16 mg/ kg/d for children <16 years

| Mullen et al. The AIMS trial ISRCTN 90011794 (United Kingdom) | Randomized, DB Irbesartan vs placebo | Sep 2010–Mar 2017 | 5 years | 490 | 6–40 years | <45 mm | Irbesartan 300 mg for patients >50 kg and 150 mg if <50 kg | Placebo |
| Forteza et al. LO-AT-MARFAN NCT 01145612 (Spain) | Randomized, DB Losartan vs Atenolol | Oct 2008–Feb 2013 | 3 years | 150 | 5–60 years | <45 mm | Losartan 2.5 mg/day for patients <50 kg or 25 mg/day for patients >50 kg (14 days). From day 15:50 mg/day or 25 mg/day for patients <50 kg | Atenolol 12.5 mg/day for patients <50 kg or 25 mg/day for patients >50 kg (14 days). From day 15:50 mg/day or 25 me/day for patients <50 kg |

(continued)

TABLE 4.4 (continued)

First author (country)	Name and identification number	Study design and objectives	Year trial started – estimated completion	Follow-up	Estimated enrolment	Age	Aortic size at entry	Drug and daily dosage	Control drug and daily dosage
Radonic et al. (Netherlands)	COMPARE study NTR 1423	Randomized, open-label Losartan vs not-treated controls	Feb 2008– Feb 2010	3 years	330	≥18 years	Aortic root diameter <50 mm	Losartan 50 mg (first 14 days) or 100 mg (after first 14 days)	Patients taking β-blockers will continue their treatment
Chiu et al. (Taiwan)	NCT 00651235	Randomized, open-label Losartan added to β-blockers	Feb 2007– Feb 2011	3 years	44	≥1 year	Z-score >2	Losartan 100 mg/day for adults and 50 mg/day for children. Atenolol 50 mg/day; Propranolol 20 mg/twice daily for adults, 1 mg/kg/day for children	Atenolol or Propranolol. Atenolol or Propranolol is 150 mg/ day for adult and 2 mg/kg/day for children

Möberg et al. (Belgium)	NCT 00782327	Randomized, DB Losartan added to β-blockers vs placebo	June 2009– Dec 2014	3 years	174	>10 years Z-score ≥2		Losartan 50 mg for <50 kg and 100 mg if >50 kg	Placebo
Creager et al. (USA)	NCT 00723801	Randomized, DB Losartan vs Atenolol on aortic stiffness	Oct 2007– Dec 2012	6 months	50	>25 years	ND	Losartan 100 mg/day	Atenolol 50 mg/day
Sander et al. (Canada)	NCT 00593710	Randomized, DB Losartan vs Atenolol on aortic PWV	Jan 2008– Dec 2011	12 months	30	12–25 years	ND	Losartan 25 mg/day	Atenolol 25–50 mg/ day

NCT ClinicalTrials.gov number, *ISRCTN* International Standard Randomised Controlled Trial Number, *NTR* Netherlands Trial Register, *PWV* pulse wave velocity, *SB* single-blind, *DB* double-blind, *ND* not described betablocker used in the USA trial (atenolol). Its vasodilator properties could reduce the rebound wave and therefore the stress applied on the proximal aorta and enhance the haemodynamic benefit of the drug; its beta-1 selectivity should increase its tolerance and therefore compliance. Finally, the relative benefits of the two classes of drug and their combination are ideal. The drawback of having three groups is the need for a high number of patients (n: 291) to obtain the statistical power necessary to recognise differences between groups.

The *University of Ghent trial* [88] has a design similar to the French trial, but also evaluates the evolution of aortic stiffness over time. The objective is to include 174 MFS patients (age ≥ 10 years and z-score ≥ 2). Patients already taking β-blockers are randomised for weight-adjusted treatment with losartan versus placebo. The primary end-point is to reduce the aortic root growth rate. MRI evaluation will be made at baseline and at the end of the trial. The similar design may permit a secondary combination of the populations to increase statistical power, which is obviously an issue when the protocol aims to include such a selected population.

The English *AIMS* [89] (Aortic Irbesartan Marfan Study) Trial is studying the effects of another ARB, irbesartan, in Marfan patients. For this study, 490 Marfan patients (aged ≥ 6 and ≤40) will be enrolled and randomised to 2 groups: irbesartan vs. placebo. The therapeutic dose of ARB will be uptitrated to the maximum tolerated dose in 2 months (target dose 300 mg/die for patients ≥50 kg, 150 mg/die if <50 kg) and continued for 5 years. Patients with previous cardiac or aortic surgery are excluded. The primary outcome of that multicentre, prospective, randomised, double-blind trial will be evaluation of the different rate of aortic root dilatation between these groups measured by transthoracic echocardiography. Annual echocardiography follow-up will be carried out. Importantly, standard medical treatment (including β-blockers) will be given to all patients, if tolerated. Therefore, the study is not designed to evaluate the effects of irbesartan monotherapy in MSF, but rather the effects of combined therapy. However, analysis of β-blocker-intolerant patient subgroup could also permit estimation of the effects of irbesartan alone.

The Spanish trial is a clinical trial conducted at two institutions. One hundred and fifty subjects of both sexes diagnosed with MFS, aged between 5 and 60 years, and who meet the Ghent diagnostic criteria will be included in the study, with 75 patients per treatment group. It will be a randomised, double-blind trial with parallel assignment to atenolol or losartan (50 mg per day in patients under 50 kg and 100 mg per day in patients over 50 kg). Both growth and distensibility of the aorta will be assessed with echocardiography and magnetic resonance. Follow-up will be 3 years.

Special Conditions

Medical Treatment in Operated Patients

After ascending aorta surgery, the distal aorta is still susceptible to dilatation or dissection [90]; thus, close imaging follow-up is required in these patients. Furthermore, the maintenance of long-term treatment with β-blockers and exercise restrictions must also be considered. A subgroup analysis from the COMPARE trial [82] suggested that the addition of losartan was significantly associated with a reduced dilatation rate of the aortic arch. However, this result should be interpreted with caution as baseline aortic dimensions in patients with prior aortic root replacement were not completely comparable between the treatment groups.

Medical Treatment in Pregnant Women

ACEI and ARB are contraindicated during pregnancy owing to the increased risk of fetal loss and birth defects. These deleterious effects have been confirmed in animal studies. Women of childbearing age under these treatments should be informed of the potential teratogenic and fetotoxic risks of these drugs if they become pregnant [91]. Data related to the use of β-blockers during pregnancy are limited. All studies are observational and retrospective. Although β-blockers have been related to a higher risk of fetal growth retardation, consensus holds that β-blockers may be used during pregnancy to prevent aortic complications [92]. However, we recommend balancing the risk-benefit ratio in each individual patient, and fetal growth should be monitored if treatment with β-blockers is prescribed. A recent retrospective observational study [93] included 29 pregnancies in 21 women with MFS and compared them with 116 controls. Mean aortic root diameter pre-pregnancy was 39.5 ± 1.3 mm in the nulliparous group (n = 21). Although the study does not compare the outcome of Marfan patients with and without β-blocker treatment, it is informative of the outcome of Marfan pregnancies under this treatment since almost all patients were taking β-blockers throughout pregnancy (n = 26; 89.7 %). In this study, there were no maternal or perinatal deaths, but complications were more likely in the MFS group. Maternal complications occurred in five pregnancies (17 %) and included one type A aortic dissection, 2 aortic surgeries within 6 months of delivery and 2 patients who developed left ventricular dysfunction. Neonates in the Marfan group were more likely to be small for gestational age.

Omnes et al. [94] also published an observational retrospective study on 22 pregnancies with maternal mean aortic root at baseline 39.0 ± 3.9 mm. Again in this study, almost all patients were under β-blocker treatment (n = 19; 86.4 %). In this cohort, aortic diameter did not increase significantly during pregnancy, one aortic dissection occurred and fetal growth restriction was observed in 7 (31.8 %) pregnancies.

In 1995, Pyeritz et al. [95] published an observational study that included 28 pregnancies in Marfan patients. In that study, only 10 patients received β-blockers, but no comparison was made between both Marfan patient groups. Two patients suffered an aortic dissection: one was not treated with β-blockers and the other did receive them.

The risk of aortic dissection in Marfan patients during pregnancy has also been related to aortic dimensions. However, there is not a completely safe aortic dimension: Marfan patients with normal aortic root diameter (generally considered <40 mm) have a low risk of aortic dissection or other cardiac complications during pregnancy [96]. ESC guidelines for cardiovascular diseases during pregnancy recommend using the WHO classification to assess maternal risk in pregnant woman with cardiovascular conditions [92]. Thus, Marfan patients with normal aortic root are classified as having a WHO II risk [97] (small increased risk of maternal mortality or moderate increase in morbidity), and cardiological quarterly checks are recommended. Marfan patients with a diameter >40 mm and also patients with an increase in aortic diameters throughout pregnancy have an increased risk of aortic complications. Moreover, in the presence of an aortic diameter >45 mm, pregnancy should be discouraged (WHO risk IV). In this scenario, some centres recommend aortic root surgery with a valve-sparing procedure (David's technique) prior to pregnancy, since the presence of a mechanical prosthetic aortic valve increases morbidity and mortality during pregnancy (WHO risk III: significant increased risk of maternal mortality or severe morbidity). However, after aortic surgery, patients remain at risk for aortic dissection in the distal aorta. Aortic root diameters between 40 and 45 mm in Marfan are generally classified as WHO risk III, but other risk factors for aortic dissection (indexed aortic root by body surface area >27 mm/m^2, family history of aortic dissection, rapid aortic growth, and aortic regurgitation) should also be taken in consideration. In these patients, monthly or bimonthly cardiological checks are recommended.

Current Recommendations

Although β-blocker therapy is currently recommended for all patients with MFS (American College of Cardiology Foundation/American Heart Association guidelines class I recommendation for the use of β-adrenergic– blocking drugs for all patients with Marfan syndrome to reduce the rate of aortic dilation), the evidence level is B. Several studies reported that β-blockers may not produce the desired haemodynamic effects in patients with marked aortic root dilatation with a heterogeneous response. Recently, many studies have shown that additional treatment with losartan improves the efficacy to reduce aortic root and ascending aorta dilatation. Therefore, this strategy may be applied in high-risk patients with aorta dilatation and in cases where β-blocker treatment does not reach the maximum doses due to poor tolerance or side effects. Until future therapy directed at the fibrillin-1 gene or the TGF-β axis ultimately proves most effective at preventing the aortic complications of MFS, β-blocker therapy remains the "standard of care". Losartan as monotherapy would only be justified in patients with severe bradycardia, asthma or other β-blocker contraindications. Effects of pharmacological therapy should be monitored closely during the initiation phase to ensure that heart rate goals and blood pressure management are optimal. Routine monitoring of proximal aortic size and growth rate, usually with echocardiography on an annual basis, is essential in all patients. In cases in which echo is technically inadequate and/or when aortic root diameter reaches 45 mm or surgery is indicated, cardiac magnetic resonance or computed tomography of the thoracic aorta are recommended. Future research and ongoing trials should elucidate the benefits, advantages and limitations of each drug or their combinations, taking into account individual factors such as age, aortic dilatation, risk factors or genetic mutations.

References

1. Collod-Beroud G, Le Bourdelles S, Ades L, Ala-Kokko L, Booms P, Boxer M, Child A, Comeglio P, De Paepe A, Hyland JC, Holman K, Kaitila I, Loeys B, Matyas G, Nuytinck L, Peltonen L, Rantamaki T, Robinson P, Steinmann B, Junien C, Beroud C, Boileau C. Update of the UMD-FBN1 mutation

database and creation of an FBN1 polymorphism database. Hum Mutat. 2003;22:199–208.

2. Loeys BL, Dietz HC, Braverman AC, Callewaert BL, De Backer J, Devereux RB, Hilhorst-Hofstee Y, Jondeau G, Faivre L, Milewicz DM, Pyeritz RE, Sponseller PD, Wordsworth P, De Paepe AM. The revised Ghent nosology for the Marfan syndrome. J Med Genet. 2010;47(7):476–85.

3. Gott VL, Greene PS, Alejo DE, Cameron DE, Naftel DC, Miller C, Gillinov AM, Laschinger JC, Pyeritz RE. Replacement of the aortic root in patients with Marfan's syndrome. N Engl J Med. 1999;340:1307–13.

4. Mueller GC, Stark V, Steiner K, Weil J, von Kodolitsch Y, Mir TS. The Kid-Short Marfan Score (Kid-SMS) – an easy executable risk score for suspected paediatric patients with Marfan syndrome. Acta Paediatr. 2013;102(2):e84–9.

5. Silverman DI, Burton KJ, Gray J, Bosner MS, Kouchoukos NT, Roman MJ, Boxer M, Devereux RB, Tsipouras P. Life expectancy in the Marfan syndrome. Am J Cardiol. 1995;75:157–60.

6. Pyeritz RE. Marfan syndrome: current and future clinical and genetic management of cardiovascular manifestations. Semin Thorac Cardiovasc Surg. 1993;5(1):11–6.

7. Murdoch JL, Walker BA, Halpern BL, Kuzma JW, McKusick VA. Life expectancy and causes of death in the Marfan syndrome. N Engl J Med. 1972;286:804–8.

8. Finkbohner R, Johnston D, Crawford ES, Coselli J, Milewicz DM. Marfan syndrome: long-term survival and complications after aortic aneurysm repair. Circulation. 1995;91:728–33.

9. Roman MJ, Rosen SE, Kramer-Fox R, Devereux RB. Prognostic significance of the pattern of aortic root dilation in the Marfan syndrome. J Am Coll Cardiol. 1993;22:1470–6.

10. Davies RR, Goldstein LJ, Coady MA, Tittle SL, Rizzo JA, Kopf GS, Elefteriades JA. Yearly rupture or dissection rates for thoracic aortic aneurysms: simple prediction based on size. Ann Thorac Surg. 2002;73:17–28.

11. Svensson LG, Kim KH, Blackstone EH, Rajeswaran J, Gillinov AM, Mihaljevic T, Griffin BP, Grimm R, Stewart WJ, Hammer DF, Lytle BW. Bicuspid aortic valve surgery with proactive ascending aorta repair. J Thorac Cardiovasc Surg. 2011;142(3): 622–9, 629.e1–3.

12. Svensson LG, Khitin L. Aortic cross-sectional area/height ratio timing of aortic surgery in asymptomatic patients with Marfan syndrome. J Thorac Cardiovasc Surg. 2002;123(2):360–1.

13. Silverman DI, Gray J, Roman MJ, Bridges A, Burton K, Boxer M, Devereux RB, Tsipouras P. Family history of severe cardiovascular disease in Marfan syndrome is associated with increased aortic diameter and decreased survival. J Am Coll Cardiol. 1995; 26:1062–7.

14. Nollen GJ, Groenink M, Tijssen JG, Van Der Wall EE, Mulder BJ. Aortic stiffness and diameter predict progressive aortic dilatation in patients with Marfan syndrome. Eur Heart J. 2004;25(13):1146–52.

15. Mortensen K, Aydin MA, Rybczynski M, Baulmann J, Schahidi NA, Kean G, Kühne K, Bernhardt AM, Franzen O, Mir T, Habermann C, Koschyk D, Ventura R, Willems S, Robinson PN, Berger J, Reichenspurner H, Meinertz T, von Kodolitsch Y. Augmentation index relates to progression of aortic disease in adults with Marfan syndrome. Am J Hypertens. 2009;22(9):971–9.

16. Yetman AT, Bornemeier RA, McCrindle BW. Long-term outcome in patients with Marfan syndrome: is aortic dissection the only cause of sudden death? J Am Coll Cardiol. 2003;41:329–32.

17. Bunton TE, Biery NJ, Myers L, Gayraud B, Ramirez F, Dietz HC. Phenotypic alteration of vascular smooth muscle cells precedes elastolysis in a mouse model of Marfan syndrome. Circ Res. 2001;88:37–43.

18. Booms P, Pregla R, Ney A, Barthel F, Reinhardt DP, Pletschacher A, Mundlos S, Robinson PN. RGD-containing fibrillin-1 fragments upregulate matrix metalloproteinase expression in cell culture: a potential factor in the pathogenesis of Marfan syndrome. Hum Genet. 2005;116:51–61.

19. Segura AM, Luna RE, Horiba K, Stetler-Stevenson WG, McAllister HA, Willerson JT, Ferrans VJ. Immunohistochemistry of matrix metalloproteinases and their inhibitors in the thoracic aortic aneurysms and aortic valves of patients with Marfan's syndrome. Circulation. 1998;98:II-331–7.

20. Neptune ER, Frischmeyer PA, Arking DE, et al. Dysregulation of TGF-beta activation contributes to pathogenesis in Marfan syndrome. Nat Genet. 2003;33(3):407–11.

21. Isogai Z, Ono RN, Ushiro S, et al. Latent transforming growth factor beta-binding protein 1 interacts with fibrillin and is a microfibril-associated protein. J Biol Chem. 2003;278:2750–7.

22. Chaudhry SS, Cain SA, Morgan A, et al. Fibrillin-1 regulates the bioavailability of TGFbeta1. J Cell Biol. 2007;176:355–67.

23. Ng CM, Cheng A, Myers LA, et al. TGF-beta-dependent pathogenesis of mitral valve prolapse in a mouse model of Marfan syndrome. J Clin Invest. 2004;114:1586–92.

24. Joint Task Force on the Management of Valvular Heart Disease of the European Society of Cardiology (ESC); European Association for Cardio-Thoracic Surgery (EACTS), Vahanian A, Alfieri O, Andreotti F, Antunes MJ, Barón-Esquivias G, Baumgartner H, Borger MA, Carrel TP, De Bonis M, Evangelista A, Falk V, Iung B, Lancellotti P, Pierard L, Price S, Schäfers HJ, Schuler G, Stepinska J, Swedberg K, Takkenberg J, Von Oppell UO, Windecker S, Zamorano JL, Zembala M. Guidelines on the management of valvular heart disease (version 2012). Eur Heart J. 2012;33(19):2451–96.

25. Hirata K, Triposkiadis F, Sparks E, Bowen J, Wooley CF, Boudoulas H. The Marfan syndrome: abnormal aortic elastic properties. J Am Coll Cardiol. 1991;18(1):57–63.

26. Kiotsekoglou A, Moggridge JC, Kapetanakis V, Newey VR, Kourliouros A, Mullen MJ, Kaski JC, Nassiri DK, Camm J, Sutherland GR, Child AH. Assessment of carotid compliance using real time vascular ultrasound image analysis in Marfan syndrome. Echocardiography. 2009;26(4):441–51.

27. Kiotsekoglou A, Moggridge JC, Saha SK, Kapetanakis V, Govindan M, Alpendurada F, Mullen MJ, Camm J, Sutherland GR, Bijnens BH, Child AH. Assessment of aortic stiffness in marfan syndrome using two-dimensional and Doppler echocardiography. Echocardiography. 2011;28(1):29–37.

28. Groenink M, de Roos A, Mulder BJ, Verbeeten Jr B, Timmermans J, Zwinderman AH, Spaan JA, van der Wall EE. Biophysical properties of the normal-sized aorta in patients with Marfan syndrome: evaluation with MR flow mapping. Radiology. 2001;219(2):535–40.

29. Teixido-Tura G, Redheuil A, Rodríguez-Palomares J, Gutiérrez L, Sánchez V, Forteza A, Lima JA, García-Dorado D, Evangelista A. Aortic biomechanics by magnetic resonance: early markers of aortic disease in Marfan syndrome regardless of aortic dilatation? Int J Cardiol. 2014 ;171(1):56–61.

30. Laurent S, Cockcroft J, Van Bortel L, Boutouyrie P, Giannattasio C, Hayoz D, Pannier B, Vlachopoulos C, Wilkinson I, Struijker-Boudier H, European Network for Non-invasive Investigation of Large Arteries. Expert consensus document on arterial stiffness: methodological issues and clinical applications. Eur Heart J. 2006;27(21):2588–605.

31. Halpern BL, Char F, Murdoch JL, Horton WB, McKusick VA. A prospectus on the prevention of aortic rupture in the Marfan syndrome with data on survivorship without treatment. Johns Hopkins Med J. 1971;129:123–9.

32. Ose L, McKusick VA. Prophylactic use of propranolol in the Marfan syndrome to prevent aortic dissection. Birth Defects. 1977;13:163–9.

33. Williams B, Lacy PS, Thom SM, Cruickshank K, Stanton A, Collier DV, et al.; CAFE Investigators; Anglo-Scandinavian Cardiac Outcomes Trial Investigators; CAFE Steering Committee and Writing Committee. Differential impact of blood pressure-lowering drugs on central aortic pressure and clinical outcomes: principal results of the Conduit Artery Function Evaluation (CAFE) study. Circulation. 2006;113:1213–25.

34. Jondeau G, Boutouyrie P, Lacolley P, Laloux B, Dubourg O, Bourdarias JP, Laurent S. Central pulse pressure is a major determinant of ascending aorta dilation in Marfan syndrome. Circulation. 1999;99(20):2677–81.

35. Yin FCP, Brin KP, Ting C-T, Pyeritz RE. Arterial hemodynamic indexes in Marfan's syndrome. Circulation. 1989;79:854–62.

36. Rios AS, Silber EN, Bavishi N, Varga P, Burton BK, Clark WA, et al. Effect of long-term beta-blockade on aortic root compliance in patients with Marfan syndrome. Am Heart J. 1999;137:1057–61.

37. Groenink M, DeRoos A, Mulder BJM, Spaan JAE, VanDerWall EE. Changes in aortic distensibility and pulse wave velocity assessed with magnetic resonance imaging following beta-blocker therapy in the Marfan syndrome. Am J Cardiol. 1998;82:203–8.

38. Reed CM, Fox ME, Alpert BS. Aortic biomechanical properties in paediatric patients with the Marfan syndrome, and the effects of atenolol. Am J Cardiol. 1993;71:606–8.

39. Mahmud A, Feely J. b-Blockers reduce aortic stiffness in hypertension but nebivolol, not atenolol, reduces wave reflection. Am J Hypertens. 2008;21:663–7.

40. Kampus P, Serg M, Kals J, Zagura M, Muda P, Kanu K, et al. Differential effects of nebivolol and metoprolol on central aortic pressure and left ventricular wall thickness. Hypertension. 2011;57:1122–8.

41. Cholley BP, Shroff SG, Sandelski J, Korcarz C, Balasia BA, Jain S, et al. Aortic and other vascular disease: differential effects of chronic oral antihypertensive therapies on systemic arterial circulation and ventricular energetics in African-American patients. Circulation. 1995;91:1052–62.

42. Williams A, Kenny D, Wilson D, Fagenello G, Nelson M, Dunstan F, Cockcroft J, Stuart G, Fraser AG. Effects of atenolol, perindopril and verapamil on haemodynamic and vascular function in Marfan syndrome - a randomised, double-blind, crossover trial. Eur J Clin Invest. 2012;42(8):891–9.

43. Gambarin FI, Favalli V, Serio A, Regazzi M, Pasotti M, Klersy C, et al. Rationale and design of a trial evaluating the effects of losartan vs. nebivolol vs. the association of both on the progression of aortic root dilation in Marfan syndrome with FBN1 gene mutations. J Cardiovasc Med (Hagerstown). 2009;10:354–62.

44. Habashi JP, Judge DP, Holm TM, Cohn RD, Loeys BL, Cooper TK, Myers L, Klein EC, Liu G, Calvi C, Podowski M, Neptune ER, Halushka MK, Bedja D, Gabrielson K, Rifkin DB, Carta L, Ramirez F, Huso DL, Dietz HC. Losartan, an AT1 antagonist, prevents aortic aneurysm in a mouse model of Marfan syndrome. Science. 2006;312(5770):117–21.

45. Heldin CH, Miyazono K, TenDijke P. TGF-beta signalling from cell membrane to nucleus through SMAD proteins. Nature. 1997;390:465–71.

46. Habashi JP, Doyle JJ, Holm TM, Aziz H, Schoenhoff F, Bedja D, Chen Y, Modiri AN, Judge DP, Dietz HC. Angiotensin II type 2 receptor signaling attenuates aortic aneurysm in mice through ERK antagonism. Science. 2011;332(6027):361–5.

47. Kakuta H, Sudoh K, Sasamata M, Yamagishi S. Telmisartan has the strongest binding affinity to angiotensin II type 1 receptor: comparison with other angiotensin II type 1 receptor blockers. Int J Clin Pharmacol Res. 2005;25:41–6.

48. Takagi H, Yamamoto H, Iwata K, Goto SN, Umemoto T, ALICE (All-Literature Investigation of Cardiovascular Evidence) Group. An evidence-based hypothesis for beneficial effects of telmisartan on Marfan syndrome. Int J Cardiol. 2012;158:101–2.

49. Liao JK, Laufs U. Pleiotropic effects of statins. Annu Rev Pharmacol Toxicol. 2005;45:89–118.

50. Takemoto M, Liao JK. Pleiotropic effects of 3-hydroxy-3-methylglutaryl coenzyme a reductase inhibitors. Arterioscler Thromb Vasc Biol. 2001;21(11):1712–9.

51. Chung AW, Au Yeung K, Sandor GG, Judge DP, Dietz HC, van Breemen C. Loss of elastic fiber integrity and reduction of vascular smooth muscle contraction resulting from the upregulated activities of matrix metalloproteinase-2 and −9 in the thoracic aortic aneurysm in Marfan syndrome. Circ Res. 2007;101:512–22.

52. Curci JA, Mao D, Bohner DG, Allen BT, Rubin BG, Reilly JM, Sicard GA, Thompson RW. Preoperative treatment with doxycycline reduces aortic wall expression and activation of matrix metalloproteinases in patients with abdominal aortic aneurysms. J Vasc Surg. 2000;31(2):325–42.

53. Manning MW, Cassis LA, Daugherty A. Differential effects of doxycycline, a broad-spectrum matrix metalloproteinase inhibitor, on angiotensin II-induced atherosclerosis and abdominal aortic aneurysms. Arterioscler Thromb Vasc Biol. 2003;23(3): 483–8.

54. Prall AK, Longo GM, Mayhan WG, Waltke EA, Fleckten B, Thompson RW, Baxter BT. Doxycycline in patients with abdominal aortic aneurysms and in mice: comparison of serum levels and effect on aneurysm growth in mice. J Vasc Surg. 2002;35(5): 923–9.

55. Chung AW, Yang HH, Radomski MW, van Breemen C. Long-term doxycycline is more effective than atenolol to prevent thoracic aortic aneurysm in marfan syndrome through the inhibition of matrix metalloproteinase-2 and −9. Circ Res. 2008;102(8): e73–85.

56. Guo G, Ott C, Grünhagen J, Muñoz-García B, Pletschacher A, Kallenbach K, von Kodolitsch Y, Robinson N. Indomethacin prevents the progression of thoracic aortic aneurysm in Marfan syndrome mice. Aorta. 2013;1(1):5–12.

57. Guo G, Booms P, Halushka M, Dietz HC, Ney A, Stricker S, et al. Induction of macrophage chemotaxis by aortic extracts of the mgR Marfan mouse model and a GxxPG-containing fibrillin-1 fragment. Circulation. 2006;114:1855–62.

58. Guo G, Gehle P, Doelken S, Martin-Ventura JL, von Kodolitsch Y, Hetzer R, et al. Induction of macrophage chemotaxis by aortic extracts from patients with Marfan syndrome is related to elastin binding protein. PLoS One. 2011;6:e20138.

59. Guo G, Muñoz-García B, Ott C, Grünhagen J, Shaaba A, Pletschacher A, et al. Antagonism of GxxPG fragments ameliorates manifestations of aortic disease in Marfan syndrome mice. Hum Mol Genet. 2013;22(3):433–43.

60. Ladouceur M, et al. Effect of beta-blockade on ascending aortic dilatation in children with the Marfan syndrome. Am J Cardiol. 2007;99(3):406–9.

61. Legget ME, Unger TA, O'Sullivan CK, et al. Aortic root complications in Marfan's syndrome: identification of a lower risk group. Heart. 1996;75:389–95.

62. Salim MA, Alpert BS, Ward JC, Pyeritz RE. Effect of beta-adrenergic blockade on aortic root rate of dilatation in the Marfan's syndrome. Am J Cardiol. 1994;74:629–33.

63. Selamet Tierney ES, et al. Beta-blocker therapy does not alter the rate of aortic root dilation in pediatric patients with Marfan syndrome. J Pediatr. 2007;150(77–82).

64. Yetman AT, Bornemeier RA, McCrindle BW. Usefulness of enalapril versus propranolol or atenolol for the prevention of aortic dilation in patients with the Marfan syndrome. Am J Cardiol. 2005;95:1125–7.

65. Rossi-Foulkes R, Roman MJ, Rosen SE, Kramer-Fox R, Ehlers KH, O'Loughlin JE, et al. Phenotypic features and impact of beta blocker or calcium antagonist therapy on aortic lumen size in the Marfan syndrome. Am J Cardiol. 1999;83:1364–8.

66. Shores J, Berger KR, Murphy EA, Pyeritz RE. Progression of aortic dilatation and the benefit of long-term beta-adrenergic blockade in Marfan's syndrome. N Engl J Med. 1994;33:1335–41.

67. Alpert BS, Reed CM, Ward J, Pyeritz RE, Phelps S, Bryant E. Atenolol reduces aortic growth in Marfan's syndrome (abstr). Am J Med Genet. 1993;47:143.

68. Rosen SE, Roman MJ, Kramer-Fox R, Devereux RB. The effect of chronic beta blockade therapy on aortic root dilatation in patients with Marfan's syndrome (abstr). Am J Med Genet. 1993;47:157.

69. Tahernia AC. Cardiovascular anomalies in Marfan's syndrome: the role of echocardiography and beta-blockers. South Med J. 1993;86:305–10.

70. Feingold B, Selamet S, Park SC, et al. Beta-blocker therapy does not alter aortic root growth rate in pediatric patients with Marfan's syndrome. Circulation. Suppl III 2004;110(17):#1928 (abstr).

71. Gersony DR, McClaughlin MA, Jin Z, Gersony WM. The effect of beta-blocker therapy on clinical outcome in patients with Marfan's syndrome: a meta-analysis. Int J Cardiol. 2007;114(3):303–8.

72. Hiratzka LF, Bakris GL, Beckman JA, Bersin RM, Carr VF, Casey Jr DE, Eagle KA, Hermann LK, Isselbacher EM, Kazerooni EA, Kouchoukos NT, Lytle BW, Milewicz DM, Reich DL, Sen S, Shinn JA, Svensson LG, Williams DM, American College of Cardiology Foundation/American Heart Association Task Force on Practice Guidelines; American Association for Thoracic Surgery; American College of Radiology; American Stroke Association; Society of Cardiovascular Anesthesiologists; Society for Cardiovascular Angiography and Interventions; Society of Interventional Radiology; Society of Thoracic Surgeons; Society for Vascular Medicine. 2010 ACCF/AHA/AATS/ACR/ASA/SCA/SCAI/SIR/STS/SVM guidelines for the diagnosis and management of patients with Thoracic Aortic Disease: a report of the American College of Cardiology Foundation/American Heart Association Task Force on Practice Guidelines, American Association for Thoracic Surgery,

American College of Radiology, American Stroke Association, Society of Cardiovascular Anesthesiologists, Society for Cardiovascular Angiography and Interventions, Society of Interventional Radiology, Society of Thoracic Surgeons, and Society for Vascular Medicine. Circulation. 2010;121(13): e266–369.

73. Doyle JJ, Habashi JP, Lindsay ME, Bedja D, Dietz HC. Calcium channel blockers exacerbate aortic disease and cause premature lethality in Marfan syndrome. Circulation. 2010;122, A14647.

74. Lacourciere Y, Beliveau R, Conter HS, et al. Effects of perindopril on elastic and structural properties of large arteries in essential hypertension. Can J Cardiol. 2004;20:795–9.

75. Nagashima H, Sakomura Y, Aoka Y, et al. Angiotensin 2 type receptor mediated vascular smooth muscle cell apoptosis in cystic medial degeneration associated with Marfan's syndrome. Circulation. 2001;104(Suppl I):I-282–7.

76. Nagashima H, Uto K, Sakomura Y, et al. An angiotensin-converting enzyme inhibitor, not an angiotensin 2 type 1 receptor blocker, prevents b-aminopropionitrile monofumarate-induced aortic dissection in rats. J Vasc Surg. 2002;36:818–23.

77. Ahimastos AA, Aggarwal A, D'Orsa KM, Formosa MF, White AJ, Savarirayan R, Dart AM, Kingwell BA. Effect of perindopril on large artery stiffness and aortic root diameter in patients with Marfan syndrome: a randomized controlled trial. JAMA. 2007;298(13):1539–47.

78. Schieffer B, Bunte C, Witte J, et al. Comparative effects of angiotensin-1 antagonism and angiotensin-converting enzyme inhibition on markers of inflammation and platelet aggregation in patients with coronary artery disease. J Am Coll Cardiol. 2004;44:362–8.

79. Lavoie P, Robitaille G, Agharazii M, Ledbetter S, Lebel M, Larivière R. Neutralization of transforming growth factor-beta attenuates hypertension and prevents renal injury in uremic rats. J Hypertens. 2005;23(10):1895–903.

80. Lim DS, Lutucuta S, Bachireddy P, Youker K, Evans A, Entman M, Roberts R, Marian AJ. Angiotensin II blockade reverses myocardial fibrosis in a transgenic mouse model of human hypertrophic cardiomyopathy. Circulation. 2001;103(6):789–91.

81. Brooke BS, Habashi JP, Judge DP, Patel N, Loeys B, Dietz 3rd HC. Angiotensin II blockade and aortic-root dilation in Marfan's syndrome. N Engl J Med. 2008;358(26):2787–95.

82. Groenink M, den Hartog AW, Franken R, Radonic T, de Waard V, Timmermans J, Scholte AJ, van den Berg MP, Spijkerboer AM,

Marquering HA, Zwinderman AH, Mulder BJ. Losartan reduces aortic dilatation rate in adults with Marfan syndrome: a randomized controlled trial. Eur Heart J. 2013;34(45):3491–500.

83. Pees C, Laccone F, Hagl M, Debrauwer V, Moser E, Michel-Behnke I. Usefulness of losartan on the size of the ascending aorta in an unselected cohort of children, adolescents, and young adults with Marfan syndrome. Am J Cardiol. 2013;112(9):1477–83.

84. Mueller GC, Stierle L, Stark V, Steiner K, von Kodolitsch Y, Weil J, Mir TS. Retrospective analysis of the effect of angiotensin II receptor blocker versus β-blocker on aortic root growth in paediatric patients with Marfan syndrome. Heart. 2014;100(3):214–8.

85. Chiu HH, Wu MH, Wang JK, Lu CW, Chiu SN, Chen CA, Lin MT, Hu FC. Losartan added to β-blockade therapy for aortic root dilation in Marfan syndrome: a randomized, open-label pilot study. Mayo Clin Proc. 2013;88(3):271–6.

86. Lacro RV, Dietz HC, Wruck LM, et al. Rationale and design of a randomized clinical trial of beta-blocker therapy (atenolol) versus angiotensin II receptor blocker therapy (losartan) in individuals with Marfan syndrome. Am Heart J. 2007;154:624–31.

87. Detaint D, Aegerter P, Tubach F, Hoffman I, Plauchu H, Dulac Y, Faivre LO, Delrue MA, Collignon P, Odent S, Tchitchinadze M, Bouffard C, Arnoult F, Gautier M, Boileau C, Jondeau G. Rationale and design of a randomized clinical trial (Marfan Sartan) of angiotensin II receptor blocker therapy versus placebo in individuals with Marfan syndrome. Arch Cardiovasc Dis. 2010;103(5):317–25.

88. Möberg K, De Nobele S, Devos D, Goetghebeur E, Segers P, Trachet B, Vervaet C, Renard M, Coucke P, Loeys B, De Paepe A, De Backer J. The Ghent Marfan Trial – a randomized, double-blind placebo controlled trial with losartan in Marfan patients treated with β-blockers. Int J Cardiol. 2012;157(3):354–8.

89. Mullen MJ, Flather MD, Jin XY, Newman WG, Erdem G, Gaze D, Valencia O, Banya W, Foley CE, Child A. A prospective, randomized, placebo-controlled, double-blind, multicenter study of the effects of irbesartan on aortic dilatation in Marfan syndrome (AIMS trial): study protocol. Trials. 2013;14:408.

90. Engelfriet PM, Boersma E, Tijssen JG, Bouma BJ, Mulder BJ. Beyond the root: dilatation of the distal aorta in Marfan's syndrome. Heart. 2006;92(9):1238–43.

91. Polifka JE. Is there an embryopathy associated with first-trimester exposure to angiotensin-converting enzyme inhibitors

and angiotensin receptor antagonists? A critical review of the evidence. Birth Defects Res A Clin Mol Teratol. 2012;94(8): 576–98.

92. European Society of Gynecology (ESG); Association for European Paediatric Cardiology (AEPC); German Society for Gender Medicine (DGesGM), Regitz-Zagrosek V, Blomstrom Lundqvist C, Borghi C, Cifkova R, Ferreira R, Foidart JM, Gibbs JS, Gohlke-Baerwolf C, Gorenek B, Iung B, Kirby M, Maas AH, Morais J, Nihoyannopoulos P, Pieper PG, Presbitero P, Roos-Hesselink JW, Schaufelberger M, Seeland U, Torracca L; ESC Committee for Practice Guidelines. ESC Guidelines on the management of cardiovascular diseases during pregnancy: the Task Force on the Management of Cardiovascular Diseases during Pregnancy of the European Society of Cardiology (ESC). Eur Heart J. 2011;32(24):3147–97.

93. Curry R, Gelson E, Swan L, Dob D, Babu-Narayan S, Gatzoulis M, Steer P, Johnson M. Marfan syndrome and pregnancy: maternal and neonatal outcomes. BJOG. 2014;121(5):610–7.

94. Omnes S, Jondeau G, Detaint D, Dumont A, Yazbeck C, Guglielminotti J, Luton D, Azria E. Pregnancy outcomes among women with Marfan syndrome. Int J Gynaecol Obstet. 2013;122(3): 219–23.

95. Rossiter JP, Repke JT, Morales AJ, Murphy EA, Pyeritz RE. A prospective longitudinal evaluation of pregnancy in the Marfan syndrome. Am J Obstet Gynecol. 1995;173(5):1599–606.

96. Pyeritz RE. Maternal and fetal complications of pregnancy in the Marfan syndrome. Am J Med. 1981;71:784–90.

97. Jastrow N, Meyer P, Khairy P, Mercier LA, Dore A, Marcotte F, Leduc L. Prediction of complications in pregnant women with cardiac diseases referred to a tertiary center. Int J Cardiol. 2011;151(2):209–13.

Chapter 5
Acute Aortic Syndrome: Medical Management

Christoph A. Nienaber

Introduction

Both chronic and acute diseases of the aorta, including trauma, are attracting increasing attention both in the light of an ageing Western population and with the advent of modern diagnostic modalities and therapeutic options to manage aortic pathology. In the case of aortic ectasia the individual rate of expansion and the risk of rupture may be assessed from co-morbidities, hypertensive state, or connective tissue disease, and should be quantified regardless of anatomic location for timely selection and treatment. Acute aortic syndrome, a term comprising acute dissection, intramural haematoma, and penetrating aortic ulcers, may share common ground by the observation of microapoplexy of the aortic wall, eventually leading to higher wall stress, facilitating progressive dilatation, intramural haemorrhage, dissection, and eventually rupture; chronic hypertension and connective tissue disorders are likely to promote this mechanism.

C.A. Nienaber, MD, PhD
Heart Center Rostock, University of Rostock,
Ernst-Heydemann-Str. 6, 18057 Rostock, Germany
e-mail: christoph.nienaber@med.uni-rostock.de

A. Evangelista, C.A. Nienaber (eds.), *Pharmacotherapy in Aortic Disease*, Current Cardiovascular Therapy, Vol. 7, DOI 10.1007/978-3-319-09555-4_5, © Springer International Publishing Switzerland 2015

Definition

Acute aortic syndrome (AAS) consists of different emergency conditions with similar clinical characteristics and challenges. These conditions include aortic dissection, intramural haematoma (IMH), transection following trauma and penetrating atherosclerotic ulcer (PAU). The common denominator of AAS is disruption of the media layer of the aorta with bleeding with IMH along the wall of the aorta, resulting in separation of the layers of the aorta, or transmurally through the vessel wall in case of ruptured PAU or trauma. In the majority of patients (90 %), an intimal disruption is present that results in tracking of blood between the layers of the media potentially rupturing through the adventitia or back through the intima into the aortic lumen [1]. With regards to the time domain, acute dissection is defined as occurring within 2 weeks of onset of initial pain; subacute, between 2 and 8 weeks from the onset of pain; and chronic, more than 8 weeks from the onset of pain. Anatomically, acute thoracic aortic dissection can be classified according to either the origin of the intimal tear or whether the dissection involves the ascending aorta [2]. The two most commonly used classification schemes are the DeBakey and the Stanford systems (Fig. 5.1).

Prevalence of Risk Factors

Aortic dissection and its variants are rare diseases, with an estimated incidence of approximately 2.6-3.5 cases per 100,000 person/year [3]. Around 0.5 % of patients presenting to an emergency department with chest of back pain suffer from aortic dissection [4]; two-thirds of them are male, with an average age at presentation of approximately 65 years. A history of systemic hypertension found in up to 72 % of patients is by far the most common risk factor (Table 5.1). Atherosclerosis, a history of prior cardiac surgery, and known aortic aneurysm are other major risk factors [5]. The epidemiology of aortic dissection is substantially different in young patients (<40 years of age) where risk factors such as Marfan

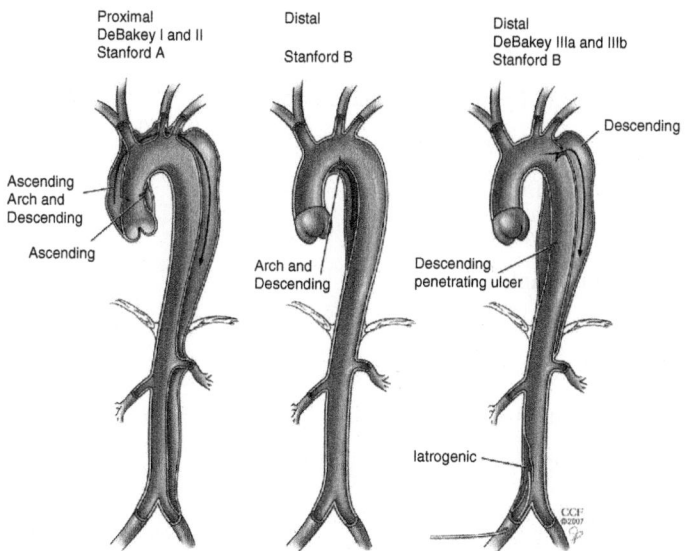

FIGURE 5.1 Aortic dissection classification: DeBakey and Stanford classification as the currently most frequently used classification systems for aortic dissection

syndrome and other connective tissue disorders take precedence. In general 60 % of aortic dissections are classified as proximal (type A) and 40 % as distal (type B) according to the Stanford classification. The PAU seems to affect mostly the descending thoracic aorta and abdominal aorta in 80 % of cases [6]. Data from previous studies suggest an incidence of PAU ranging from 2.3 to 11 % in patients presenting with AAS [7]. Conversely, acute IMH accounts for 5–20 % of all AAS; both of them have a clear relation to old age, arterial hypertension, and atherosclerosis [8].

Presentation and Diagnosis

The symptoms of an IMH with or without PAU are similar to those of acute aortic dissection. Although they are distinct pathologies, differentiation between such aortic conditions

TABLE 5.1 Risk conditions for aortic dissection

Long standing arterial hypertension
Smoking, dyslipidemia, cocaine/crack
Connective tissue disorders
Hereditary fibrillinopathies
Marfan Syndrome
Ehlers-Danlos Syndrome
Hereditary vascular disease
Bicuspid aortic disease
Coarctation
Vascular inflammation
Giant cell arteritis
Takayasu arteritis
Behcet's disease
Syphilis
Ormond's disease
Deceleration trauma
Car accident
Fall from height
Iatrogenic factors
Catheter/instrument intervention
Valvular/aortic surgery
Side or cross clamping/aortotomy
Graft anastomosis
Patch aortoplasty
Aortic wall fragility

TABLE 5.2 Demographics and history of patients with acute aortic dissection

Variable	n[a] (%)	Type A, n (%)	Type B, n (%)	P
		(N = 289)	(N = 175)	Type A vs B
Demographics				
Age, mean (SD), y	63.1 (14.0)	61.2 (14.1)	66.3 (13.2)	<0.001
Male	303 (65.3)	182 (63.0)	121 (69.1)	0.18
Patient history				
Marfan syndrome	22/449 (4.9)	19 (6.7)	3 (1.8)	0.02
Hypertension	326/452 (72.1)	194 (69.3)	132 (76.7)	0.08
Atherosclerosis	140/452 (31.0)	69 (24.4)	71 (42)	<0.001
Prior aortic dissection	29/453 (6.4)	11 (3.9)	18 (10.6)	0.005
Prior aortic aneurysm	73/453 (16.1)	35 (12.4)	4 (2.3)	0.006
Diabetes	23/451 (5.1)	12 (4.3)	11 (6.6)	0.29
Prior cardiac surgery	83 (17.9)	46 (15.9)	37 (21.1)	0.16

N = 464

[a]Denominator of reported responses is given if different than stated in the column heading

can be difficult or even impossible solely by clinical means. Patients are typically around 60 years of age with comorbidities ranging from hypertension and Marfan's syndrome to prior surgery or vascular interventions (Table 5.2). Pain is the most commonly presenting symptom of acute aortic dissection, independent of age, sex, or other associated clinical complaints [3]; pooled data from over 1,000 cases showed that acute dissection is perceived as abrupt pain in 84 % with severe intensity in 90 %. Although classically described as tearing or ripping, patients are more likely to describe the pain of acute dissection as sharp or stabbing, and fluctuating [4].

Pain location and associated symptoms reflect the site of initial intimal disruption and may change as the dissection extends along the aorta or involves other arteries or organs. Three modern imaging techniques have contributed to a better understanding of the development, natural history and diagnosis of these uncommon aortic pathologies: computerized tomographic angiography (CTA), magnetic resonance angiography (MRA), and transoesophageal echocardiography (TEE) [9–12].

Management

Initial management of AAS, particularly dissection, is directed at limiting propagation of dissected wall components by control of blood pressure and reduction in dP/dt (pressure development). Reduction in pulse pressure to just maintain sufficient end-organ perfusion is a priority with the use of intravenous β-blockade as first-line therapy [13].

Risk of Misdiagnosis

Diagnostic imaging studies in the setting of clinical suspicion of dissection have important primary goals such as confirmation of clinical suspicion, classification of dissection, localization of tears and assessment of both extent of dissection and indicators of urgency (e.g. pericardial, mediastinal, or pleural hemorrhage); in addition, biomarkers (such as myocardial markers, D-dimer elevation >500 μg/L and smooth muscle myosin heavy chain) may be used strategically in concert with swift aortic imaging, although an ideal algorithm has yet to be determined [12, 14–17]. Selection of imaging is often hospital-specific, but CT angiography is most readily available and accurate (Table 5.3). Clinical suspicion of acute aortic syndrome is high with abrupt or severe retrosternal or interscapular chest pain often migrating down the back; associated findings can produce signs of acute aortic insufficiency,

TABLE 5.3 Comparative diagnostic utility of imaging techniques in aortic dissection

	TOE	CT	MRI	Aortography
Sensitivity	++	++	+++	++
Specificity	+++	++	+++	++
Classification	+++	++	++	+
Intimal flap	+++	−	++	+
Aortic regurgitation	+++	−	++	++
Pericardial effusion	+++	++	++	−
Branch vessel involvement	+	++	++	+++
Coronary artery involvement	++	+	+	+++

pericardial effusion or occluded aortic sidebranches causing ischemia or pulse differential [4]. With predisposing factors such as hypertension, connective tissue disorders, bicuspid aortic valve, coarctation and previous cardiac surgery or recent percutaneous instrumentation, undelayed diagnostic imaging is required for any of the above symptoms and suspected acute aortic syndrome (Table 5.4) [13]. While transthoracic ultrasound provides vital information (new-onset aortic insufficiency, pericardial effusion or even visualisation of proximal dissection), additional transoesophageal (TEE) interrogation of the thoracic aorta is the logical next step, or MD-CT scanning of the entire aorta if considered safe [5, 10, 11, 17]. Both imaging modalities provide further detail beyond classification as type A and B (or distal) dissection and allow for strategic planning; ultrasound technology is portable, avoids transport of a critically-ill patient and may even be held in the operating theatre [17]. MRI has no place in the urgent diagnostic work-up of acutely symptomatic patients. Additional information not essential for immediate management decisions such as coronary, arch vessel and sidebranch involvement is usually depicted on CT-angiograms without the need for invasive angiography, even in the presence of ST-changes [5, 11].

TABLE 5.4 Management of patients with suspected aortic dissection

Recommendation	Class
ECG: documentation of ischemia	I
Heart rate and blood pressure monitoring	I
Pain relief (morphine sulfate)	I
Reduction of systolic blood pressure using beta-blockers (I.V. metoprolol, esmolol, or labetolol)	I
In patients with severe hypertension despite beta-blockers, additional vasodilator (i.v. sodium nitroprusside to titrate blood pressure to 100–120 mmHg	I
In patients with obstructive pulmonary disease, blood pressure lowering with calcium channel blockers	II
Imaging in patients with ECG signs of ischemia before thrombolysis if aortic pathology is suspected	II
Chest X-ray	III
Diagnostic Imaging (noninvasive)	I

Reproduced from Erbel et al. [40]

Medical Management

All patients must receive the best medical treatment available at admission [5, 13]. Initial management of AAS is directed at limiting propagation of diseased wall components by control of blood pressure and reduction in dP/dt. Reduction in pulse pressure with a target systolic pressure of 100–120 mmHg and a heart rate of 60–80 bpm to just maintain sufficient end-organ perfusion is a priority with the use of intravenous ß-blockade as first-line therapy. Often multiple agents are required, with patients ideally managed in an intensive care setting. Opiate analgesia should be prescribed to attenuate the sympathetic release of catecholamines to pain with resultant tachycardia and hypertension (Table 5.5). High-risk but asymptomatic patients with AAS, with the exception of type A aortic dissection, can probably be followed up without urgent intervention if they do not reveal

TABLE 5.5 Initial medical treatment in patients with acute aortic dissection and hypertension

Name	Mechanism	Dose	Cautions/contraindications
Esmolol	Cardioselective beta-1 blocker	Load: 500 µg/kg IV	Asthma or bronchospasm
		Drip: 50 µg kg⁻¹ min⁻¹ IV.	Bradycardia
		Increase by increments of 50 µg/min	2nd- or 3rd-degree AV block
			Cocaine or methamphetamine abuse
Labetalol	Nonselective beta 1,2 blocker	Load: 20 mg IV	Asthma or bronchospasm
	Selective alpha-1 blocker	Drip: 2 mg/min IV	Bradycardia
			2nd or 3rd degree AV block
			Cocaine or methamphetamine abuse
Enalaprilat	ACE inhibitor	0.625–1.25 mg IV q 6 h.	Angioedema
		Max dose: 5 mg q 6 h.	Pregnancy
			Renal artery stenosis

(continued)

TABLE 5.5 (continued)

Name	Mechanism	Dose	Cautions/contraindications
Nitroprusside	Direct arterial vasodilator	Begin at 0.3 µg kg^{-1} min^{-1} IV.	Severe renal insufficiency
			May cause reflex tachycardia
		Max dose 10 µg kg^{-1} min^{-1}	Cyanide/thiocyanate toxicity – especially in renal or hepatic insufficiency
Nitroglycerin	Vascular smooth muscle relaxation	5–200 µg/min IV	Decreases preload – contraindicated in tamponade or other preload-dependent states
			Concomitant use of sildenafil or similar agents

any early complications [2, 18, 19]. All symptomatic patients will need surgical or interventional treatment, since the evolution is unpredictable with a high likelihood of severe complications. Moreover, it is clearly necessary to distinguish IMH and PAU from classic acute aortic dissection. The site of lesion and evidence of complications, as well as evidence of disease progression on serial imaging dictate the management strategy besides the initial medical management.

Control of Pain

First-line therapy is pain relief by morphine sulphate and intravenous β-blockade. The use of benzodiazepines and labetalol, with both α- and β-blockade, is useful for lowering both blood pressure and dP/dt, with target systolic pressure of 100–120 mmHg and heart rate of 60–80 beats/min. Often multiple agents are required, with patients ideally managed in an intensive care setting. Opiate analgesia should be prescribed to attenuate the sympathetic release of catecholamines to pain with resultant tachycardia and hypertension. Further management is dictated by the site of the lesion and evidence of complications (persisting pain, organ malperfusion), as well as evidence of disease progression on serial imaging.

Control of Blood Pressure

On admission, any AAS patient is subject to standardised protocol management including ICU transfer, continuous arterial pressure monitoring, central venous access for administration of intravenous antihypertensive agents, and urine output monitoring via a bladder catheter. The initial goals are to halt progression of dissection by decreasing impulse force (of systolic pressure) and control pain; β-blocking agent (labetalol, metoprolol), calcium channel blockers, nitroglycerine and sodium nitroprusside are used in that order to ensure anti-impulse management with the goal of keeping blood pressure <120 mmHg and mean arterial pressure

<80 mmHg. Patients remain in cardiovascular intensive care until pressure and pain are well controlled and medication is oralised. In presence of uncontrollable pain or pressure elevation, evidence of a complicated setting of type B dissection is likely and endovascular management is usually warranted; the spectrum of complicated type B dissection is widening with ongoing pain and hypertension as recent, but nevertheless, classic complications [13, 20, 21]. There is no evidence for endovascular repair of uncomplicated type B dissection with no ongoing symptoms and well-controlled blood pressure and no evidence of malperfusion or impending rupture. The INSTEAD trial showed no survival advantage of stenting as opposed to best medical therapy at 2 years (best medical therapy 95.6 % vs. stenting 88.9 %; P = 0.15) [22] The study, however, showed a beneficial impact of stent-graft on aortic remodelling and beneficial long-term outcomes [23–25].

Management of Complications

In the case of suspected aortic dissection, prompt and competent interpretation of diagnostic contrast-enhanced CT or other imaging is mandatory for undelayed triaging and proper treatment. A high clinical index of suspicion after a "negative" result from the initial diagnostic imaging study may warrant subsequent transoesophageal ultrasound interrogation at the bedside. Moreover, focused cardiac ultrasound (FOCUS) can be useful for time-sensitive rapid assessment of aortic root size, valvular function and presence of dissection or intramural haematoma. Beyond transthoracic evaluation, transoesophageal imaging offers clear depiction of both ascending and descending aorta at high temporal resolution with clear depiction of entry size and location, secondary communications, extra-aortic blood collection and of true lumen collapse or compression; such information has a major prognostic impact and identifies patients at risk for ongoing or impending complications. As a consequence, all features of aortic wall disintegration or dissection involving the ascending aorta requires immediate surgical attention or prompt transfer to an appropriate tertiary care centre. Conversely, with features of complications such as impending rupture or organ malperfusion including true lumen collapse, type B dissection also requires undelayed attention by use of endovascular technology to reconstruct the true lumen of the dissected aorta. In particular, in presence of shock symptoms, the assumption of a scenario of complicated dissection is highly likely either caused by loss of blood by rupture, by hypotension secondary to bowel ischaemia from malperfusion and obstruction of the superior mesenteric artery and/or the celiar trunk. Similarly, but not as acutely, the emergence of renal dysfunction may be due to proximal aortic true lumen collapse or bilateral renal artery obstruction from dissection, and of course, requires endovascular revascularisation procedures, along with immediate volume expansion and fluid hydration.

Shock

Shock with diagnostic confirmation of a type A dissection (or any aortic pathology involving the ascending aorta) should prompt undelayed surgery and open repair. Cardiogenic shock is either caused by pericardial tamponade (frequent with proximal dissection), by acute aortic valve regurgitation or by coronary compromise from the dissection lamella either progressing into the left coronary mainstem or just obstructing any coronary ostium or from rare other conditions (Table 5.6). Interventions such as pericardiocentesis or coronary percutaneous procedures are not advised because they can worsen the acute problem and cost precious time until life-saving surgery. Shock from acute blood loss indicates rupture or contained rupture of the aorta and the need for immediate surgery, but is often fatal.

In a type B setting, shock symptoms call for immediate volume expansion (including blood transfusion) and swift endovascular management of such a life-threatening complication in an attempt to seal major communications to the

TABLE 5.6 Clinical findings in aortic dissection

Hypotension or shock due to:

  (a) Hemopericardium and pericardial tamponade

  (b) Acute aortic insufficiency due to dilatation of the aortic annulus

  (c) Aortic rupture

  (d) Lactic acidosis

  (e) Spinal shock

Acute myocardial ischemia/infarction due to coronary ostial occlusion

Pericardial friction rub due to hemopericardium

Syncope

Pleural effusion or frank hemothorax

Acute renal failure due to dissection across renal arteries

Mesenteric ischemia due to dissection across intra-abdominal arteries

Neurologic deficits:

  (a) Stroke due to occlusion of arch vessels

  (b) Limb weakness

  (c) Spinal cord deficits due to cord ischemia

  (d) Hoarseness due to compression of left recurrent laryngeal nerve

false lumen and thereby stop further blood loss via the ruptured outer media layer of the false lumen.

Renal Insufficiency

In the setting of both proximal and also distal dissection, acute renal insufficiency can be the result of kidney malperfusion from obstructed renal arteries. The obstruction often results from true lumen collapse or from static obstruction of renal arteries by either thrombus or invagination of dissected aortic wall components. In most cases, local interventions are not helpful and would delay urgent proximal repair in type A dissection; in type B dissection, malperfusion of renal arteries are best managed by endovascular scaffolding of the descending thoracic aorta with stent-graft in the true lumen, an intervention that depressurises the false lumen, redirects blood to the true lumen only, and opens the true lumen by virtue of systolic pressure even at the level of abdominal side branches and iliac arteries. After such a procedure, stents in the ostia of renal arteries are rarely needed and fenestration procedures are obsolete. Renal function usually recovers even after days of malperfusion.

Anticoagulation

Risk/Benefit of Anticoagulation and Antithrombotics

Once a proximal or distal aortic dissection has been diagnosed, therapeutic management is focused on surgical repair in cases of type A involvement and on proper triaging for complications and thus endovascular treatment of type B dissection. There is no place for anticoagulation strategies besides the use of prophylactic heparin to avoid deep venous thrombosis during immobilisation and bed rest. With ambulation, patients do not require anticoagulants either in the short term, or long-term. Similarly, no antiaggregation with agents such as aspirin or thienopyridiues is required except for unrelated independent indications such as coronary or peripheral artery disease. Even after TEVAR, specific antithrombotic medication is not indicated. On the other hand, chronic dissection without signs of acute complications is not a contraindication for antithrombotic or anticoagulant medication if they are needed for another prognostically relevant reason [2].

Interventional Management

In the acute setting with complications, endovascular repair for dissection of the descending thoracic aorta is now established owing to the high mortality of open repair [2, 21, 26]. Conversely, open surgical repair requires single-lung ventilation, cardiopulmonary bypass with circulatory arrest, profound hypothermia and cerebrospinal fluid drainage, and has been replaced by endovascular repair with an IA recommendation in the presence of organ or limb ischemia [27–29]. Particularly in the setting of malperfusion, outcomes with open surgery have been unpredictable and the risk of irreversible spinal cord injury and death in acute type B dissections has ranged from 14 to 67 % [2, 3, 30]. Contemporary in-hospital mortality rates are around 17 % with open surgery supporting a paradigm shift towards endovascular management as first-line treatment in patients with complicated type B dissection [21, 31, 32]. If malperfusion of a branch vessel persists, branch vessel stenting or the PETTICOAT (provisional extension to induce complete attachment) technique may be used with open bare-metal stents to relieve distal malperfusion [33, 34] (Fig. 5.2). In complex complicated scenarios, even the interventional closure of distal re-entry points appears reasonable with successful endovascular management the 30-day mortality of 10.8 % for complicated dissection with imminent rupture or end organ ischemia is similar to the mortality rate of uncomplicated patients [29]. Nevertheless, complications can occur with TEVAR including peri-intervention stroke and retrograde dissection particularly in inexperienced hands [35]. A relatively dated meta-analysis of outcomes for TEVAR in complicated acute type B aortic dissection, revealed in-hospital mortality of 9 %, and a low rate of major complications (stroke 3.1 %; paraplegia 1.9 %; conversion to type A dissection 2 %; bowel infarction 0.9 %; and major amputation 0.2 %); aortic rupture occurred in 0.8 % over 20 months concluding that endovascular treatment of (complicated) acute type B dissection is a therapeutic option with favourable initial outcomes; the

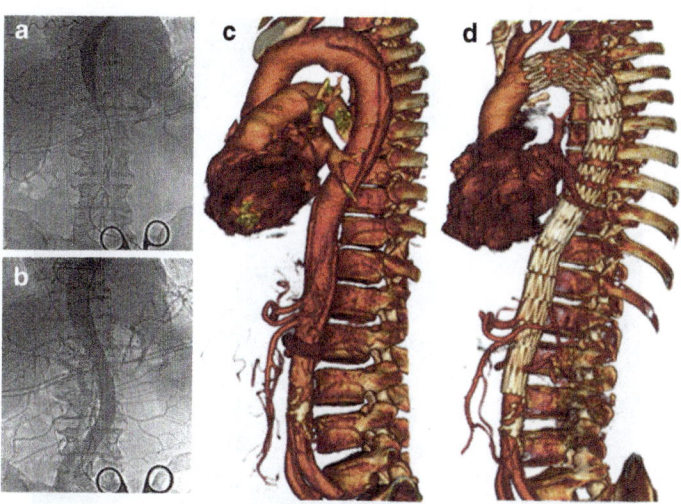

FIGURE 5.2 Malperfusion syndrome treated with endovascular stent-graft and PETTICOAT; (**a**) angiography of lower body malperfusion; (**b**) reperfusion after proximal stent-graft; (**c**) 3D CT reconstruction of acute complicated dissection with malperfusion; (**d**) reconstructed aorta and abolished malperfusion after stent-graft and PETTICOAT

long-term data regarding outcome and remodelling are promising [28]. Current observational evidence suggests that TEVAR improves survival in complicated distal dissection [21]. In patients with connective tissue disease, however, remodeling is achieved less frequently and endovascular strategies are discouraged or considered as bridging to definitive open repair [36].

In the subacute phase of distal aortic dissection, mortality varies between 32 % for open surgery, 7 % for patients with endovascular management, and 10 % for medical treatment alone (P<0.0001) [3, 32]. Approximately 60 % of late deaths result from rupture of the false lumen since long-term patency of the false lumen sets the stage for aneurysmal dilatation (Fig. 5.3). Previously accepted indications for surgical repair, such as refractory pain, ongoing malperfusion,

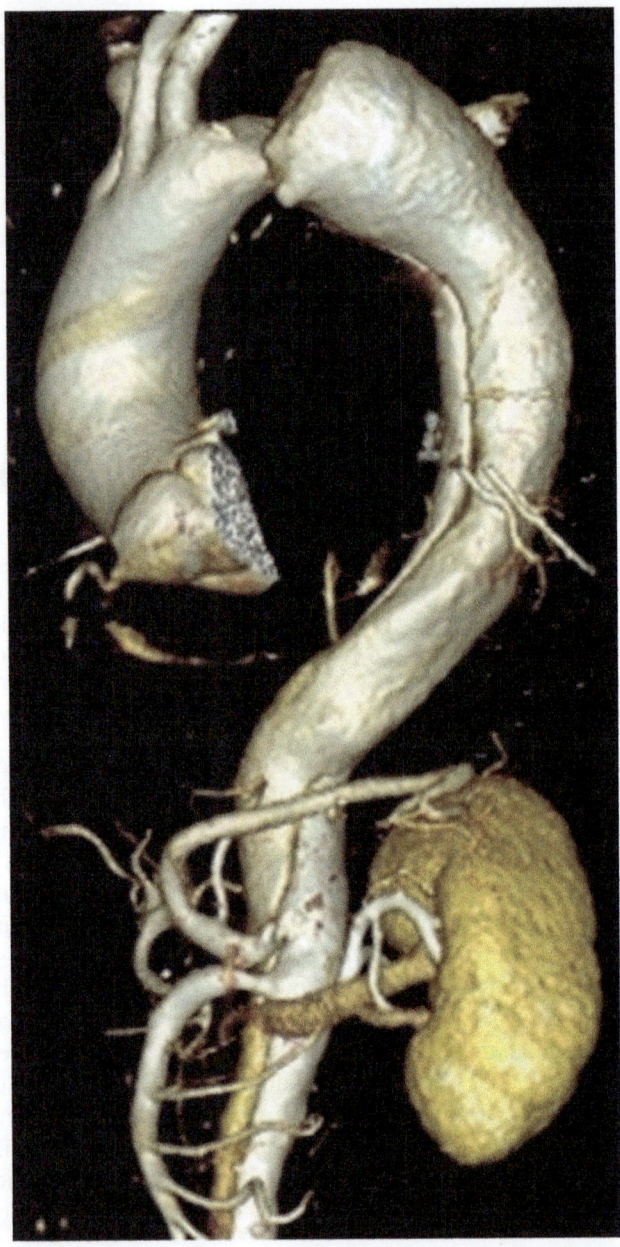

FIGURE 5.3 3D-CT image of aneurysmal dilatation of uncomplicated type B aortic dissection after 3 years

expansion >1 cm per year, and a diameter over 55 mm are currently considered indications for TEVAR in subacute and chronic dissections. There is clear observational evidence that depressurisation and shrinkage of the false lumen are beneficial even beyond the acute phase of dissection, and placement of an individualised stentgraft has been shown to promote false lumen thrombosis and remodelling even late after dissection. Stent-graft placement has even been used to treat late evolution of retrograde extension into the ascending aorta, followed by remodelling and healing in a subacute state. This window of plasticity of dissected aorta is usually open until 90 days; in other words, the likelihood of successful remodelling with TEVAR is greater in the first 3 months than later in the chronic phase of dissection [26].

Surprisingly, the only randomised comparison demonstrated no statistical difference in all-cause mortality between patients treated with TEVAR compared with best medical therapy alone for up to 2 years of follow-up [22]. However, long-term outcome data support endovascular scaffolding (with stent-graft) for initially stable type B dissection in an attempt to prevent late complications and cardiovascular death [23, 24, 37]; therefore, in concert with antihypertensive medication, pre-emptive TEVAR provided at low risk is increasingly being accepted even for initially uncomplicated dissection [23, 37]. At 5 years of follow-up the INSTEAD-XL study showed that aortic rupture, disease progression and vascular mortality to be tempered by pre-emptive TEVAR in the sub-acute phase of dissection (Fig. 5.4). The pre-emptive TEVAR concept, as introduced above in the subacute phase of dissection, is supported by one meta-analysis and 2 retrospective registries [23, 37]; in particular observations from IRAD corroborate the late advantage of TEVAR beyond 2–3 years of follow-up [24]. Thus, anatomically-suitable patients with considerable life expectancy of >2 years should be offered pre-emptive TEVAR regardless of clinical presentation with the idea to prevent late complications. Such a conceptual change from a complication-specific indication for TEVAR to pre-emptive TEVAR also suggests that patients with dissection should be transferred to tertiary care at high-volume aortic centres for high-quality care and at a very low complication rate [38].

Outlook

Different clinical patterns are being used to differentiate between sets of patients with aortic dissection, both in type A but, in particular, in type B. While management of type A dissection is straightforward with the need for timely surgical repair after initial pain control and blood pressure control by intravenous drugs, subclassification of type B dissections is more complex although all type B dissections represent a serious

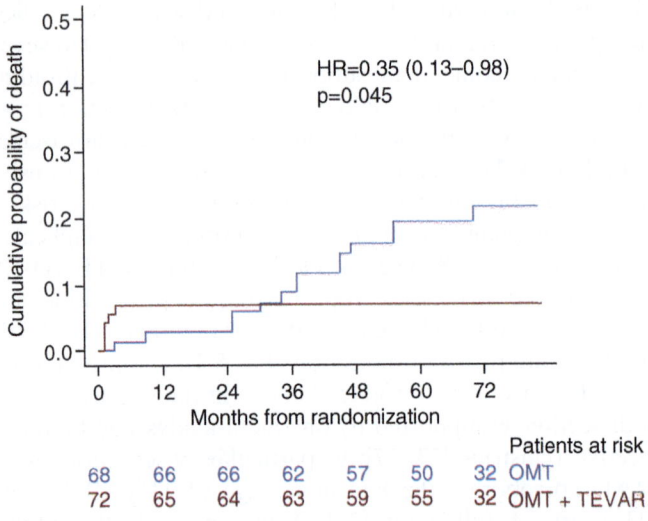

FIGURE 5.4 Five years F/U INSTEAD-XL vascular mortality. Kaplan-Meier estimates of vascular mortality (death), and landmark analysis with the breakpoint at 24 month, 12 month and 1 month after randomization to the end of the trial are shown for OMT and OMT+TEVAR groups. Beyond 2 years of follow-up the observed mortality was lower with TEVAR than with OMT alone [23]

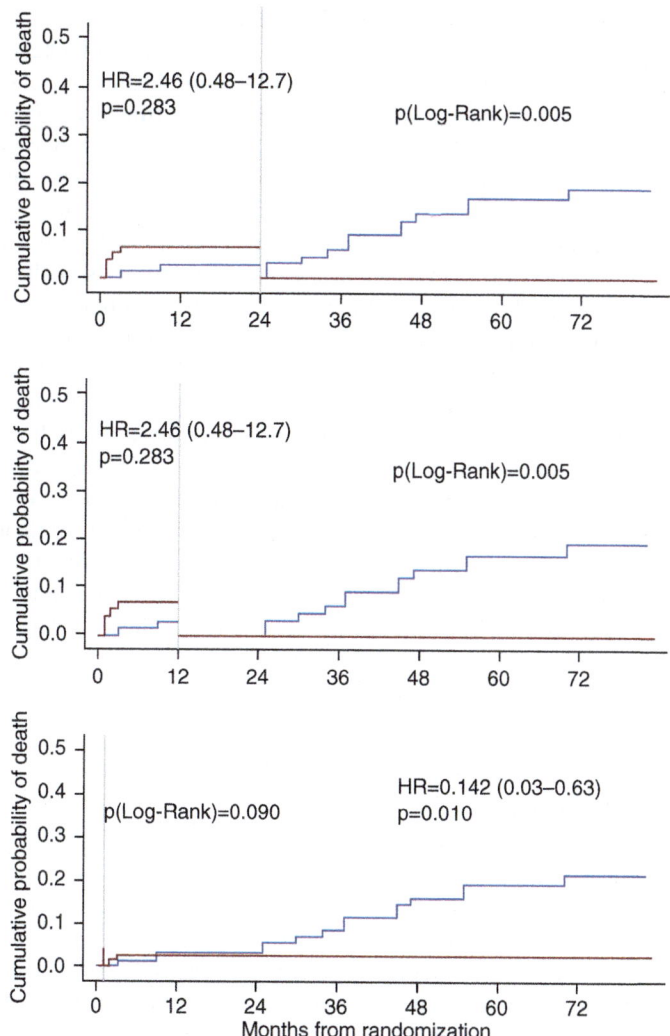

FIGURE 5.4 (continued)

vascular event per se as the result of longstanding uncontrolled hypertension, connective tissue disorders or other risk conditions with the potential to shorten lifespan. Currently used recommendations suggest initial medical management (anti-impulse β-blockade, sartans and/or Ca^{++}-channel blockers) with close surveillance for so-called uncomplicated type B dissections in the acute, subacute and chronic setting; emergent TEVAR is accepted and advised in all complicated scenarios of type B dissection. This complication-driven approach may soon be supplanted by a more liberal pre-emptive use of TEVAR (with advanced technology) in the light of long-term benefits from aortic remodeling, even in the setting of so-called uncomplicated type B dissection. Thus, with better understanding of adverse predictors, the concept of pre-emptive repair of any type B aortic dissection by endovascular interventions should be considered for all patients with type B dissection regardless of presenting symptoms and in addition to life-long pharmaceutical blood pressure control as long as they are anatomically suitable. All patients should be followed and offered sustained surveillance with focus on blood pressure control and progressive expansion; even renal sympathetic denervation may have a role [39]. With this novel approach, chances are that thoraco-abdominal aneurysmatic expansion of dissected aortas could be prevented in the future.

Intramural Haematoma and Penetrating Aortic Ulcer

Medical management of intramural haematoma and penetrating aortic ulcer follows the same logic as aortic dissection. In type A involvement, surgery should be considered in all cases except in presence of serious comorbidities. Before surgery or in cases where surgery is not indicated, medical treatment including control of symptoms and haemodynamic alterations is indicated.

In type B involvement, management is based on complications. In cases without complications, control of pain and blood pressure are paramount. Repeated imaging during the acute phase is necessary to monitor evolution of intramural or periaortic haemorrhage, progression of aorta size and disease extension.

References

1. Ledbetter S, Stuk JL, Kaufman JA. Helical (spiral) CT in the evaluation of emergent thoracic aortic syndromes: traumatic aortic rupture, aortic aneurysm, aortic dissection, intramural hematoma, and penetrating atherosclerotic ulcer. Radiol Clin North Am. 1999;37:575–89.

2. Hiratzka LF, Bakris GL, Beckman JA, et al. 2010 ACCF/AHA/AATS/ACR/ASA/SCA/SCAI/SIR/STS/SVM guidelines for the diagnosis and management of patients with thoracic aortic disease: executive summary. A report of the American College of Cardiology Foundation/American Heart Association Task Force on Practice Guidelines, American Association for Thoracic Surgery, American College of Radiology, American Stroke Association, Society of Cardiovascular Anesthesiologists, Society for Cardiovascular Angiography and Interventions, Society of Interventional Radiology, Society of Thoracic Surgeons, and Society for Vascular Medicine. Catheter Cardiovasc Interv. 2010;76(2):E43–86.

3. Hagan PG, Nienaber CA, Isselbacher EM, et al. The International Registry of Acute Aortic Dissection (IRAD): new insights into an old disease. JAMA. 2000;283(7):897–903.

4. Kodolitsch Y, Schwartz AG, Nienaber CA. Clinical prediction of acute aortic dissection. Arch Intern Med. 2000;160:2977–82.

5. Nienaber CA, Eagle KA. Aortic dissection: new frontiers in diagnosis and management. Circulation. 2003;108:628–35.

6. Coady MA, Rizzo JA, Hammond GL, et al. Penetrating ulcer of the thoracic aorta: what is it? How do we recognize it? How do we manage it? J Vasc Surg. 1998;27:1006–15.

7. Brinster DR. Endovascular repair of descending thoracic aorta for penetrating atherosclerotic ulcer of the aorta. Br J Surg. 2001;88:1169–77.

8. Evangelista A, Dominguez R, Sebastia C, et al. Long-term follow-up of aortic intramural hematoma: predictors of outcome. Circulation. 2003;108(5):583–9.

9. Nienaber CA, von Kodolitsch Y, Nicolas V, Siglow V, Piepho A, Brockhoff C, Koschyk DH, Spielmann RP. The diagnosis of thoracic aortic dissection by noninvasive imaging procedures. N Engl J Med. 1993;328(1):1–9.

10. Shiga T, Wajima Z, Apfel CC, Inoue T, Ohe Y. Diagnostic accuracy of transesophageal echocardiography, helical computed tomography, and magnetic resonance imaging for suspected thoracic aortic dissection: systematic review and meta-analysis. Arch Intern Med. 2006;166:1350–6.

11. Moore AG, Eagle KA, Bruckman D, Moon BS, Malouf JF, Fattori R, Evangelista A, Isselbacher EM, Suzuki T, Nienaber CA, Gilon D, Oh JK. Choice of computed tomography, transesophageal echocardiography, magnetic resonance imaging, and aortography in acute aortic dissection: International Registry of Acute Aortic Dissection (IRAD). Am J Cardiol. 2002;89(10):1235–8.

12. Nienaber CA, Kische S, Skriabina V, Ince H. Noninvasive imaging approaches to evaluate the patient with known or suspected aortic disease. Circ Cardiovasc Imaging. 2009;2:499–506.

13. Nienaber CA, Powell JT. Management of acute aortic syndromes. Eur Heart J. 2012;33:26–35.

14. Suzuki T, Distante A, Zizza A, Trimarchi S, Villani M, Salerno Uriarte JA, De Luca Tupputi Schinosa L, Renzulli A, Sabino F, Nowak R, Birkhahn R, Hollander JE, Counselman F, Vijayendran R, Bossone E, Eagle K, IRAD-Bio Investigators. Diagnosis of acute aortic dissection by D-dimer: the International Registry of Acute Aortic Dissection Substudy on Biomarkers (IRAD-Bio) experience. Circulation. 2009;119:2702–7.

15. Eggebrecht H, Naber CK, Bruch C, Kroger K, von Birgelen C, Schmermund A, Wichert M, Bartel T, Mann K, Erbel R. Value of plasma fibrin D-dimers for detection of acute aortic dissection. J Am Coll Cardiol. 2004;44:804–9.

16. Penco M, Paparoni S, Diagianti A, Fusilli C, Vitarelli A, De Remigis F, Mazzola A, Di Luzio V, Greogorini R, D'Eusanio G. Usefulness of transesophageal echocardiography in the assessment of aortic dissection. Am J Cardiol. 2000;86:53–6.

17. Meredith EL, Masani MD. Echocardiography in the emergency assessment of acute aortic syndromes. Eur J Echocardiogr. 2009; 10:i31–9.

18. Nienaber CA, Eagle KA. Aortic dissection: new frontiers in diagnosis and management: part II: therapeutic management and follow-up. Circulation. 2003;108(6):772–8.

19. Nienaber CA, von Kodolitsch Y, Petersen B, et al. Intramural hemorrhage of the thoracic aorta. Diagnostic and therapeutic implications. Circulation. 1995;92:1465–72.

20. Trimarchi S, Eagle KA, Nienaber CA, Pyeritz RE, Jonker FH, Suzuki T, O'Gara PT, Froehlich JB, Cooper JV, Montgomery D, Meinhardt G, Myrmel T, Upchurch GR, Sundt TM, Isselbacher EM. Importance of refractory pain and hypertension in acute type B aortic dissection: insights from the International Registry of Acute Aortic Dissection (IRAD). Circulation. 2010;122: 1283–9.

21. Nienaber CA, Kische S, Ince H, Fattori R. Thoracic endovascular aneurysm repair for complicated type B aortic dissection. J Vasc Surg. 2011;54(5):1529–33.

22. Nienaber CA, Rousseau H, Eggebrecht H, et al. INSTEAD Trial. Randomized comparison of strategies for type B aortic dissection: the INvestigation of STEnt Grafts in Aortic Dissection (INSTEAD) trial. Circulation. 2009;120:2519–28.

23. Nienaber CA, Kische S, Rousseau H, et al. Endovascular repair of type B aortic dissection: long-term results of the randomized investigation of stent grafts in aortic dissection trial. Circ Cardiovasc Interv. 2013;6(4):407–16.

24. Fattori R, Montgomery D, Lovato L, et al. Survival after endovascular therapy in patients with type B aortic dissection: a report from the International Registry of Acute Aortic Dissection (IRAD). JACC Cardiovasc Interv. 2013;6(8):876–82.

25. Ulug P, McCaslin JE, Stansby G, Powell JT. Endovascular versus conventional medical treatment for uncomplicated chronic type B aortic dissection. Cochrane Database Syst Rev. 2012;(11): CD006512.

26. Akin I, Kische S, Ince H, Nienaber CA. Indication, timing and results of endovascular treatment of type B dissection. Eur J Vasc Endovasc Surg. 2009;37:289–96.

27. Trimarchi S, Nienaber CA, Rampoldi V, et al. Role and results of surgery in acute type B aortic dissection: insights from the International Registry of Acute Aortic Dissection (IRAD). Circulation. 2006;114(1 Suppl):I357–64.

28. Parker JD, Golledge J. Outcome of endovascular treatment of acute type B aortic dissection. Ann Thorac Surg. 2008;86(5):1707–12.

29. White RA, Miller DC, Criado FJ, et al. Report on the results of thoracic endovascular aortic repair for acute, complicated, type B aortic dissection at 30 days and 1 year from a multidisciplinary subcommittee of the Society for Vascular Surgery Outcomes Committee. J Vasc Surg. 2011;53(4):1082–90.

30. Safi HJ, Estrera AL, Miller CC, et al. Evolution of risk for neurologic deficit after descending and thoracoabdominal aortic repair. Ann Thorac Surg. 2005;80(6):2173–9; discussion 9.

31. Wilkinson DA, Patel HJ, Williams DM, Dasika NL, Deeb GM. Early open and endovascular thoracic aortic repair for complicated type B aortic dissection. Ann Thorac Surg. 2013; 96(1):23–30.

32. Fattori R, Tsai TT, Myrmel T, et al. Complicated acute type B dissection: is surgery still the best option?: a report from the

International Registry of Acute Aortic Dissection. J Am Coll Cardiol Intv. 2008;1(4):395–402.

33. Nienaber CA, Kische S, Zeller T, Rehders TC, Schneider H, Lorenzen B, Bünger C, Ince H. Provisional extension to induce complete attachment after stent-graft placement in type B aortic dissection: the PETTICOAT concept. J Endovasc Ther. 2006; 13(6):738–46.

34. Canaud L, Patterson BO, Peach G, Hinchliffe R, Loftus I, Thompson MM. Systematic review of outcomes of combined proximal stent grafting with distal bare stenting for management of aortic dissection. J Thorac Cardiovasc Surg. 2013;145(6):1431–8.

35. Ullery BW, McGarvey M, Cheung AT, et al. Vascular distribution of stroke and its relationship to perioperative mortality and neurologic outcome after thoracic endovascular aortic repair. J Vasc Surg. 2012;56(6):1510–7.

36. Marcheix B, Rousseau H, Bongard V, et al. Stent grafting of dissected descending aorta in patients with Marfan's syndrome: mid-term results. J Am Coll Cardiol Intv. 2008;1(6):673–80.

37. Patterson B, Holt P, Nienaber C, Cambria R, Fairman R, Thompson M. Aortic pathology determines midterm outcome after endovascular repair of the thoracic aorta: report from the Medtronic Thoracic Endovascular Registry (MOTHER) database. Circulation. 2013;127(1):24–32.

38. Chikwe J, Cavallaro P, Itagaki S, Seigerman M, Diluozzo G, Adams DH. National outcomes in acute aortic dissection: influence of surgeon and institutional volume on operative mortality. Ann Thorac Surg. 2013;95(5):1563–9.

39. Divchev D, Turan G, Rehders T, Nienaber CA. Renal sympathetic denervation in patients with aortic dissection. J Interv Cardiol. 2014;27(3):334–9.

40. Erbel R, Alfonso F, Boileau C, et al. Task Force on Aortic Dissection of the European Society of Cardiology. Diagnosis and management of aortic dissection. Eur Heart J. 2001;22: 1642–81.

Chapter 6
Medical Treatment in Chronic Aortic Dissection

Eduardo Bossone, Francesco Ferrara, and Rodolfo Citro

Introduction

Acute aortic syndrome (AAS) is a life-threatening disease which includes classic acute aortic dissection, intramural haematoma and penetrating atherosclerotic aortic ulcer (trauma of the aorta may also be considered) sharing common physiopathological mechanisms (disruption of media), clinical characteristics and therapeutic challenges [1, 2].

Thoracic aortic dissections may be classified anatomically according to the origin of the intimal tear (DeBakey System) or whether the dissection involves the ascending aorta regardless the site of origin (Stanford System) [2] (Fig. 6.1, 6.2, and 6.3). Furthermore, it is termed acute when presentation occurs within 2 weeks, sub-acute within 2–6 weeks, and chronic more than 6 weeks after symptom onset [1].

Given the high risk of complications and non-specific symptoms and signs AAS requires a high clinical index of suspicion. Prompt diagnosis and appropriate therapeutic

E. Bossone, MD, PhD, FCCP, FESC, FACC (☒)
F. Ferrara, MD, PhD • R. Citro, MD, PhD
Heart Department, University Hospital "Scuola Medica Salernitana", Salerno, Italy
e-mail: ebossone@hotmail.com

A. Evangelista, C.A. Nienaber (eds.), *Pharmacotherapy in Aortic Disease*, Current Cardiovascular Therapy, Vol. 7, DOI 10.1007/978-3-319-09555-4_6,
© Springer International Publishing Switzerland 2015

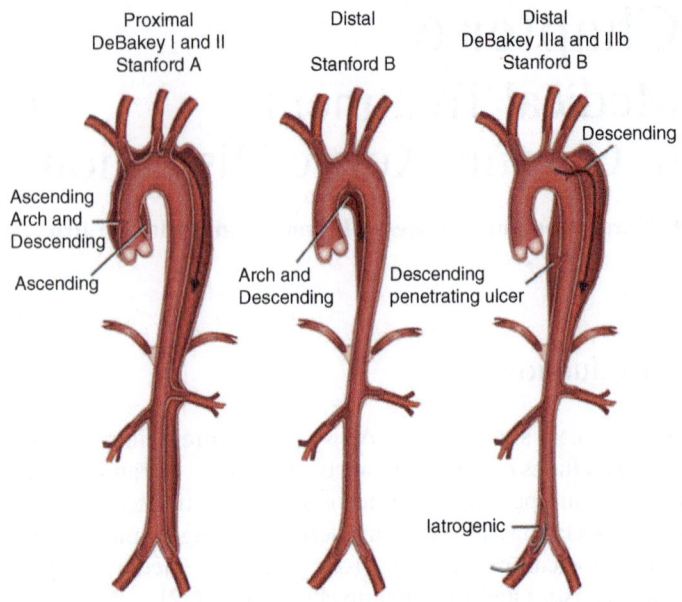

FIGURE 6.1 DeBakey and Stanford classification of aortic dissection. The DeBakey classification system categorizes dissections based on the origin of the intimal tear and the extent of the dissection: *Type I*: Dissection originates in the ascending aorta and propagates distally to include at least the aortic arch and typically the descending aorta. *Type II*: Dissection originates in and is confined to the ascending aorta. *Type III*: Dissection originates in the descending aorta and propagates most often distally. *Type IIIa*: Limited to the descending thoracic aorta. *Type IIIb*: Extending below the diaphragm. The Stanford classification system divides dissections into two categories, those that involve the ascending aorta and those that do not. *Type A*: All dissections involving the ascending aorta regardless of the site of origin. *Type B*: All dissections that do not involve the ascending aorta. Note involvement of the aortic arch without involvement of the ascending aorta in the Stanford classification is labeled as Type B (Reproduced with permission from Nienaber et al. [1])

interventions are paramount to enhance survival [1, 3]. However, after the acute phase, AAS persist with a high risk of re-dissection, aneurysm formation, and/or rupture.

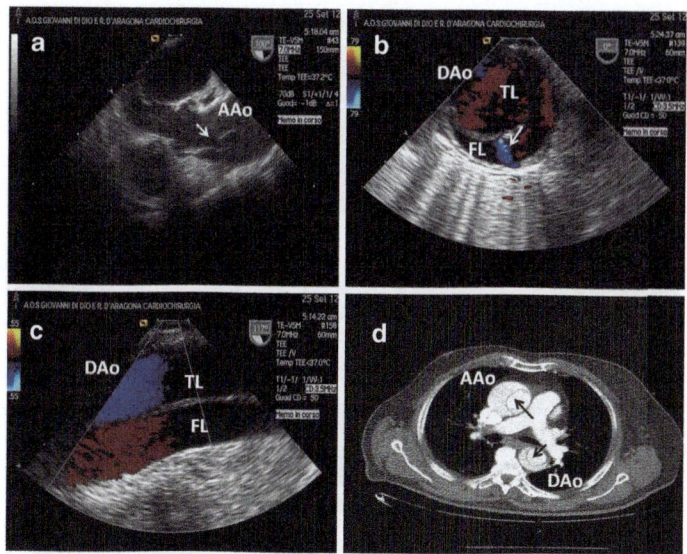

FIGURE 6.2 Chronic Stanford A aortic dissection in 68 years old man with history of hypertension and chest pain occurred 2 months before hospital admission. (**a**) Transesophageal echocardiography (TEE) in long axis view demonstrating intimal flap (see *arrow*) in ascending aorta (*AAo*). (**b**) and (**c**) TEE in short and long axis view respectively of the descending aorta (*DAo*) showing anterior true lumen (*TL*) and posterior false lumen (*FL*); note a distal small intimal tear (**b**, see *arrow*). (**d**) Computed tomography of the aorta: intimal flap (see *black arrows*) in both ascending and descending tract can be appreciated

Long-Term Outcomes

The 10-year survival rate of patients with an aortic dissection may range from 30 to 60 % [1, 4–14]. Among 303 consecutive cases with TA-AAD enrolled in the International Registry of Acute Aortic Dissection (IRAD) (90.1 % managed surgically vs 9.9 % medically), survival for patients treated with surgery was 96.1 % +2.4 % and 90.5 % ±3.9 % at 1 and 3 years versus 88.6 % ±2.2 % and 68.7 % ±19.8 % without surgery (mean follow-up overall, 2.8 years) [12] (Fig. 6.4).

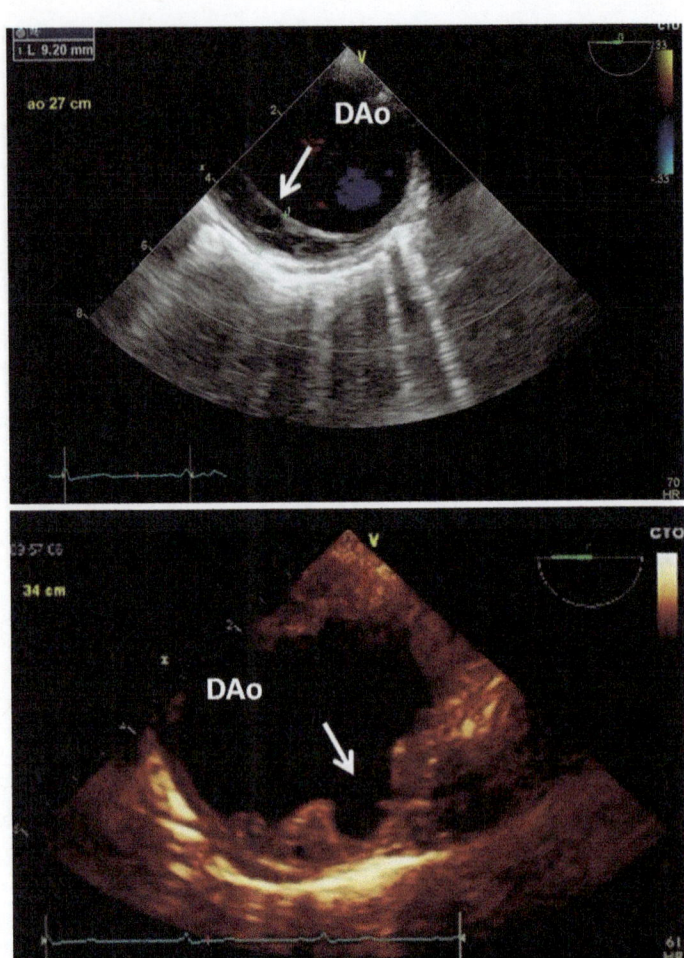

FIGURE 6.3 *Top*: TEE short axis view of the DAo. Note the abnormal thickness of posterior wall do to chronic intramural haematoma. *Bottom*: Penetrating ulcer of atherosclerotic plaque can be clearly appreciated as an incidental finding in a patient with history of hypertension and diabetes mellitus

History of atherosclerosis and previous cardiac surgery were identified as independent predictors of follow-up mortality [12]. On the other hand, 3-year survival for type B aortic

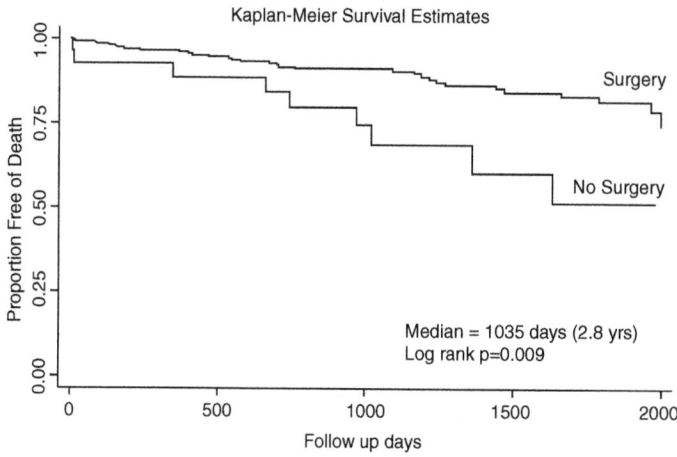

FIGURE 6.4 Unadjusted Kaplan-Meier survival curve stratified by in-hospital management from date of hospital discharge. This figure shows the survival curves estimated by the Kaplan-Meier method stratified by in-hospital management. The unadjusted survival rate at 1 year was 96.1 % ± 2.4 % and 88.6 % ± 12.2 % for surgery versus medical treatment, respectively, with further separation of the curves at 3 years with survival rates of 90.5 % ± 3.9 and 68.7 % ± 19.8 (median 2.8 years, log rank P = 0.009) (Reproduced with permission from Tsai et al. [12])

dissection patients (n = 242) treated medically, surgically, or with endovascular therapy was 77.6 ± 6.6 %, 82.8 ± 18.9 %, and 76.2 ± 25.2 %, respectively (median follow-up 2.3 years) [13] (Fig. 6.5). In that series, independent predictors of follow-up mortality included female sex, history of aortic aneurysm, history of atherosclerosis, in-hospital renal failure, pleural effusion on chest radiograph, and in-hospital hypotension/shock [13]. Some clinical predictors of complications, such as Marfan syndrome [15–17], age [17, 18], chronic obstructive pulmonary disease [17] or atherosclerotic disease have been reported [19]. In addition, maximum descending aorta diameter [12, 17, 20–22], true lumen compression or large false lumen diameter, partial false lumen thrombosis and the presence of a large proximal entry tear [23] are predictors of mortality and the need for surgical/endovascular treatment.

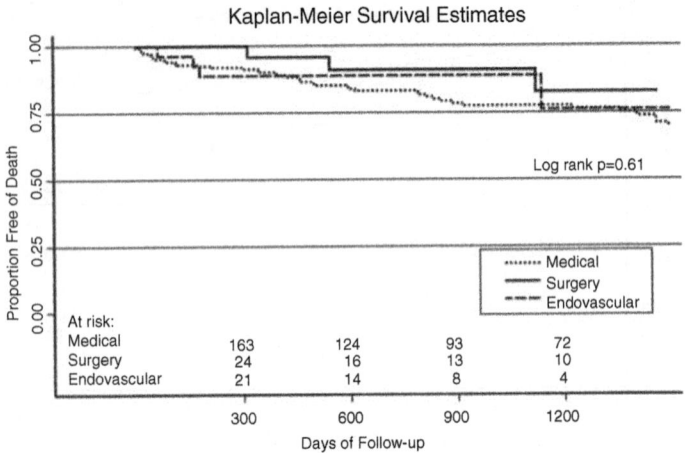

FIGURE 6.5 Unadjusted Kaplan-Meier survival curve stratified by in-hospital management. This figure shows the survival curves estimated by the Kaplan-Meier method stratified by in-hospital management. The unadjusted survival rate at 1 and 3 years for patients discharged from the hospital alive was 90.3 ± 4.3 % and 77.6 ± 6.6 % for medical therapy alone, 95.8 ± 8.0 % and 82.8 ± 18.9 % for surgery, and 88.9 ± 11.9 % and 76.2 ± 25.2 % for endovascular treatment (median 2.3 years, log-rank $P = 0.63$) (Reproduced with permission from Tsai et al. [13])

Patent false lumen in descending aorta segments after surgical treatment of type A dissection is frequent (64–90 %) [18, 24, 25]. Suboptimal connection of the distal part of the graft implanted in ascending aorta to the true lumen or presence of secondary tears may account for the persistence of flow into the distal residual false lumen after complete surgical resection of the primary entry tear. Long-term outcome of aortic dissection with patent false lumen in descending aorta presents a higher risk of complications in type B than in type A dissections, particularly after 3 years of evolution. The expansion rate of the chronic dissected aorta is not particularly well characterised, but ranges between 0.1 and 0.7 cm per year.

Evangelista et al. investigated the long-term clinical and morphological evolution of 50 IMH. In the first 6 months, total IMH regression was observed in 14 and progression to aortic

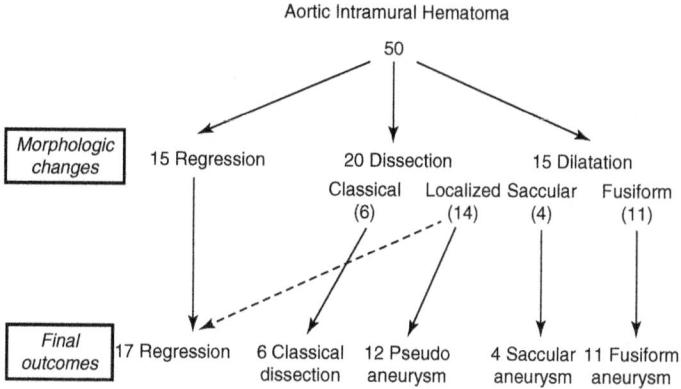

FIGURE 6.6 Different evolution patterns of IMH from morphological changes to final outcomes (Reproduced with permission from Evangelista et al. [14])

dissection in 18 patients; in 14 of these, the dissection was localised, and 12 later developed pseudoaneurysm. At the end of follow-up (mean: 45 ± 31 months), the IMH had regressed completely without dilatation in 17 patients (34 %), progressed to classical dissection in 6 (12 %), evolved to fusiform aneurysm in 11 (22 %), evolved to saccular aneurysm in 4 (8 %), and evolved to pseudoaneurysm in 12 (24 %) [14] (Fig. 6.6). Multivariate analysis showed an independent association between regression and smaller maximum aortic diameter and between aneurysm formation and atherosclerotic ulcerated plaque and absence of echolucent areas in IMH [14].

After discharge, all AAS patients need close clinical and imaging follow-up and excellent blood pressure control (minimise aortic wall stress) along with specific life style recommendations in order to prevent major complications [2, 26, 27].

Imaging Surveillance

The patient with AAD demands careful clinical and imaging monitoring by a specialised aorta team in order to detect signs of aortic expansion/dissection, aneurysm formation,

TABLE 6.1 Relative strengths of imaging modalities for acute aortic syndromes

	TTE	TEE	MRI	CT
Imaging factors				
Comprehensive aortic assessment	+	++	+++	+++
Tomographic (3D reconstruction)	–	–	+++	+++
Functional	+++	+++	++	+
Tissue characterization	–	–	+++	+++
Clinical factors				
Portability	+++	++	–	–
Patient access/monitoring	+++	+++	+	++
Rapidity	++	++	++	+++
Non-contrast	+++	+++	+	+
Radiation exposure	+++	+++	+++	+

leakages at anastomosis/stent sites, and malperfusion [2, 28]. Computed tomography (CT) and magnetic resonance imaging (MRI) providing a comprehensive evaluation of the aorta represent ideal tools for serial imaging [2, 26] (Table 6.1).

MRI, although not widely available, should be considered the technique of choice. In fact, it provides tomographic-3D reconstruction, tissue characterisation and functional assessment. It entails no radiation exposure and minimises the risk associated with the use of gadolinium – based contrast agents (excellent safety profiles). However, gadolinium-based contrast agents are contraindicated in patients with advanced renal impairment (glomerular filtration rate <30 mL/min) owing to risks of nephrogenic systemic fibrosis. MRI is prohibited in patients with ferromagnetic and/or magnetically-activated implants (including most cardiac pacemakers, defibrillators) and image artifact can interfere with the assessment of vascular stents [26–29].

Current guidelines recommend: (a) regular outpatient visits and imaging at 1, 3, 6, 9 and 12 months post-dissection and

TABLE 6.2 Imaging follow-up of aortic pathologies after repair or treatment

Pathology	Interval	Study
Acute dissection	Before discharge, 1 month, 6 months, yearly	CT or MR, chest plus abdomen TTE
Chronic dissection	Before discharge, 1 year, 2 to 3 years	CT or MR, chest plus abdomen TTE
Aorticroot repair	Before discharge, yearly	TTE
AVR plus ascending	Before discharge, yearly	TTE
Aorticarch	Before discharge, 1 year, 2 to 3 years	CT or MR, chest plus abdomen
Thoracicaortic stent	Before discharge, 1 month, 2 months, 6 months, yearly or 30 days[a]	CXR, CT, chest plus abdomen
Acute IMH/ PAU	Before discharge, 1 month, 3 months, 6 months, yearly	CT or MR, chest plus abdomen

Adapted from Erbel et al. [27]
AVR indicates aortic valve replacement, *CT* computed tomographic imaging, *CXR* chest x-ray, *IMH* intramural hematoma, *MR* magnetic resonance imaging, *PAU* penetrating atherosclerotic ulcer, *TTE* transthoracic echocardiography
[a]US Food and Drug Administration stent graft studies usually required before discharge or at 30-day CT scan to detect endovascular leaks. If there is concern about a leak, a predischarge study is recommended; however, the risk of renal injury should be borne in mind. All patients should be receiving beta blockers after surgery or medically managed aortic dissection, if tolerated

annually thereafter, depending on aortic size and the patient's clinical condition (hypertension and aortic expansion/dissection are common early after discharge), and (b) to utilise for each patient the same modality at the same institution so that similar images can be compared side by side [2, 27] (Table 6.2).

Studies have suggested detection of increased FDG uptake (marker of active inflammation) by positron emission tomography (PET)/CT may help to differentiate acute from chronic AAD. The combination of PET/CT and vascular/aortic biomarkers that reflect remodelling (e.g. transforming growth factor α [TGF-α]) may have potential risk prediction value during the following of AAS patients [30–32]. In addition, plasma MMP levels might also be used in long-term follow-up to monitor aortic remodelling [30, 33]. However, further studies are needed to explore potential clinical applications of biomarkers in chronic aortic dissection [30].

Medical Treatment (Table 6.3)

Optimal Blood Pressure Control

Hypertension represents one of the key causative factors of AAS [2, 34]. Patients with AAS often require the combination of at least two drugs to achieve blood pressure and heart rate control [35]. On the basis of the data from patients with Marfan's syndrome, long-term beta blockade (negative inotropic and chronotropic effects, lower blood pressure and decreased dp/dt) is usually recommended in patients with aortic dissection to maintain blood < 120/80 mmHg and heart rate < 60 bpm (first line) [2, 36–39]. Genoni et al. reported improved survival in patients treated with beta-blockers 1685 in the chronic phase of aortic dissection [40]. That study observed an 80 % freedom from aortic events at a mean of 4.2 years in patients on beta-blockers, in comparison with 47 % freedom from aortic events in patients treated with other anti-hypertensive agents. The efficacy of other antihypertensive drugs has not been demonstrated in patients with chronic type B aortic dissection although they have a role in maintaining the patient's blood pressure at the appropriate level. Long-acting rather than short acting beta-blockers should be preferred to reduce side effects and increase compliance. Observational studies suggest similar or better benefits in aortic dissection when compared with other antihypertensive agents [11, 41]. Guidelines recommend progressive uptitration

TABLE 6.3 Medical treatment and lifestyle goals in the follow-up of patients with chronic aortic syndrome [2]

Medical treatment

1. Optimal blood pressure < 120/80 mmHg and heart rate < 60 bpm control

   First line: beta-blockers

   Second line: ACE inhibitors or ARB

   Third line: calcium channel blockers (long-acting dihydropyridine)

2. Lipid lowering therapy: target of LDL cholesterol less than 70 mg/dL

Lifestyle goals

   Low-fat and low-salt diet

   Achieve an ideal body weight

   Smoking cessation (special programs, and/or pharmacotherapy, including nicotine, replacement, buproprion, or varenicline may be useful)

   Avoid cocaine or other stimulating drugs such as methamphetamine

   Avoid strenuous physical activities, isometric exercise, pushing, or straining that would require a Valsalva maneuver

   Avoid contact sports that can cause sudden stress or trauma to the thorax, (e.g. competitive football, ice hockey, or soccer etc.)

   Mild aerobic exercise and daily activities are not restricted

   Adherence to medical treatment

ACE angiotensin-converting enzyme inhibitors, *ARB* angiotensin receptor blockers

of dosage to achieve a blood pressure 135/80 mmHg in usual patients and 130/80 mmHg in those with Marfan syndrome [42, 43], Several studies have suggested that between 40 and 70 % of late deaths in patients with chronic aortic dissection are non-aorta related and due to comorbid diseases, mainly heart disease and stroke [15, 44], thus implying that cardiovascular risk factors should be thoroughly assessed in this group. Interestingly, cigarette smoking seems not to affect the expansion and rupture rate of chronic type B aortic dissection, although its detrimental role in cardiovascular risk is well established. Although their role in the incidence of late aortic complications has not been demonstrated, cardiovascular risk-reduction measures (such as cholesterol treatment, antiplatelet therapy, management of hypertension and smoking cessation) is advisable for patients with chronic dissections to reduce the incidence of late cardiovascular death.

Shores et al. among 70 adolescent/adult patients with classic Marfan syndrome [32 treated with propanolol vs 38 untreated (control), open label randomised trial] demonstrated that the mean slope of the regression line for the aortic root dimensions which reflect the rate of dilatation was significantly lower in the beta-blocker group than in the control group (0.023 vs. 0.084 per year, $p < 0.001$; average of 10 years follow-up) [37] (Fig. 6.7). Furthermore, long-term use of β-blockers appears to be associated with reduced progression of aortic dilatation, incidence of hospital admissions, as well as incidence of late dissection-related aortic procedures in acute type B aortic dissection patients [11, 40–45].

Additional (not optimal control) or alternative (betablocker intolerance) agents for blood pressure control are ACE inhibitors and angiotensin receptor blockers (second line) [46]. In this regard, Groenink et al. [47] among 233 adults (47 % female) with MFS [multicentre, open-label, randomised controlled trial to either losartan (n = 116) or no additional treatment (n = 117)] demonstrated that losartan treatment reduced the aortic root dilatation rate (as assessed by MRI) after 3 years of follow-up. Following prophylactic aortic root replacement, losartan treatment reduced the dilatation rate of the aortic arch [47]. Ahimastos AA et al., in a randomised, double-blind, placebo-controlled trial of 17 patients with Marfan syndrome [8 mg/day of perindopril (n = 10) or placebo (n = 7) for 24 weeks in adjunct to standard beta – blocker therapy], showed that perindopril reduced

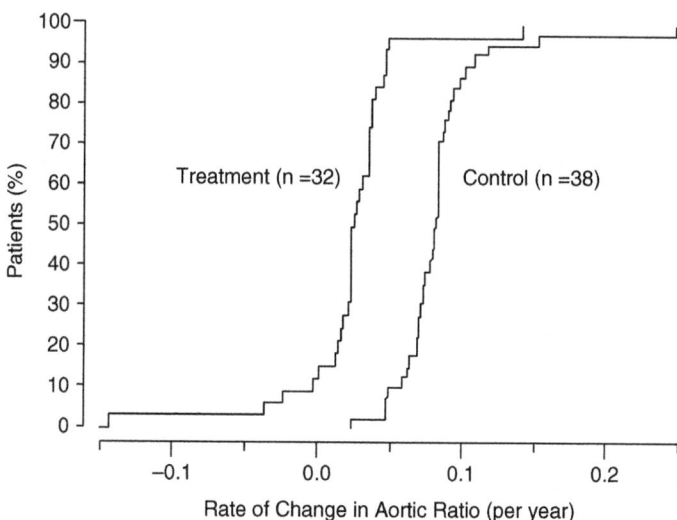

FIGURE 6.7 Empirical distribution functions of the rate of change in the aortic ratio, according to Study Group. The height of each curve at any point shows the proportion of patients with values at or below the value given on the x axis. There is little overlap between the two groups (Reproduced with permission from Shores et al. [37])

both aortic stiffness and aortic root diameter possibly through attenuation of TGF-signalling [48].

Long-acting CCB (reduced reflex tachycardia compared to short-acting) may be considered in addition to an adequate beta-blockade to reach optimal blood pressure control (third line) [2, 49, 50]. Interestingly, Suzuki et al., by analysing 1,301 patients with AAD from IRAD (722 type A AAD vs 579 type B AAD, median follow-up 26.0 months, interquartile range: 12.0–48.0), showed the use of CCB to be associated with improved survival in type B patients (OR 0.55, 95 % confidence interval 0.35–0.88, p=0.01), whereas β-blockers improved outcome only in type A patients (OR 0.47, 95 % confidence interval 0.25–0.90, p=0.02) [39]. However, data need to be confirmed by RCTs to determine the effects of single medications on the long-term outcome of a different spectrum of aortic disease and define the best medical treatment [51].

Lipid-Lowering Therapy

Patients with atherosclerotic thoracic aortic disease, with or without dissection, should be considered a coronary risk equivalent and treated with statins to achieve a target of LDL cholesterol less than 70 mg/dL. In fact atherosclerosis in any non-coronary vessel significantly increases the risk of MI and stroke (greater than 20 % event rate in 10 years) [2, 52, 53].

Anticoagulation

The degree of false lumen thrombosis in type B aortic dissection or after surgical repair of acute DeBakey type I aortic dissection can predict long-term outcomes. However, there are currently no evidence-based recommendations for anticoagulation. In a retrospective observational study [54] of 136 patients with acute DeBakey type I aortic dissection who underwent surgical repair, the early-anticoagulation group had a higher proportion of completely patent false lumens and lower partial thrombosis than the no-anticoagulation group. Mean segmental aortic growth rate was significantly lower in the early-anticoagulation group than in the no-anticoagulation group (2.9 ± 1.3 and 4.5 ± 2.8 mm/year, $p = 0.01$). Overall survival and aorta-related repeat procedure-free survival were significantly better with early anticoagulation than with no anticoagulation ($p < 0.05$). However, other studies are required to confirm these results. Regarding the risk of anticoagulation in acute intramural haematoma, there is a lack of evidence since only case reports with a disparity effect have been reported [55]. Imaging techniques such as transoesophageal echocardiography or computed tomography are fundamental in the diagnosis of intramural haematoma, assessment of cardioembolic risk and in the follow-up of the evolution of intramural haematoma, which facilitates therapeutic management. Although no established recommendation exists on anticoagulation in aortic intramural haematoma, individual risk-benefit assessment of anticoagulation and follow-up with imaging techniques are essential to elect the most appropriate therapeutic management.

Lifestyle Recommendations (Table 6.3)

American Heart Association Guidelines for the diagnosis and management of thoracic aorta disease recommend for these patients clear lifestyle targets such as regular aerobic exercise, blood pressure, cholesterol and body weight control, avoid tobacco and cocaine or other stimulating drugs that may trigger aortic catastrophes. In this regard, a stepwise strategy for smoking cessation is recommended (the 5 A's are Ask, Advise, Assess, Assist, and Arrange) including a dedicated programme and specific pharmacotherapy (nicotine replacement, buproprion, or varenicline) [2, 56–60].

Isometric exercise and Valsalva manoeuvre remain contraindicated, being associated with substantial and sudden increase in mean arterial pressure as observed during the lifting of heavy weights. It is also recommended to avoid sports that may cause thoracic stress or trauma [2].

Finally, the importance of adherence to medications, especially beta-blockers and other antihypertensive drugs [2, 60], should be emphasized.

Interdisciplinary Expert Consensus for Treatment of Chronic Type B Aortic Dissection

A recent interdisciplinary expert consensus of cardiovascular, vascular and interventional specialists delineated specific recommendations and related algorithms for the treatment of acute and chronic type B aortic dissection. They confirmed that patients with uncomplicated chronic type B dissection should undergo strict blood pressure control, as stated above in to avoid false lumen dilatation and reduce wall stress [61].

On the other hand, complicated cases (defined by recurrence of symptoms, aneurysmal dilation (total aortic diameter > 55 mm) or a yearly increase (>4 mm) in aortic diameter) should be considered for TEVAR or, if contraindicated, open surgery repair. In this regard, it should underline that open surgery repair carries a higher rate of early mortality than TEVAR. Imaging surveillance and life-style goals remain key steps, irrespective of the type of therapeutic intervention.

Conclusions

Patients with AAS, regardless of the initial therapeutic interventions, deserve long term clinical monitoring by a dedicated team to include imaging surveillance, optimal blood pressure control, lipid lowering and specific life-style targets.

References

1. Nienaber CA, Powell JT. Management of acute aortic syndromes. Eur Heart J. 2012;33(1):26–35b.
2. Hiratzka LF, Bakris GL, Beckman JA, Bersin RM, Carr VF, Casey Jr DE, Eagle KA, Hermann LK, Isselbacher EM, Kazerooni EA, Kouchoukos NT, Lytle BW, Milewicz DM, Reich DL, Sen S, Shinn JA, Svensson LG, Williams DM, American College of Cardiology Foundation/American Heart Association Task Force on Practice Guidelines; American Association for Thoracic Surgery; American College of Radiology; American Stroke Association; Society of Cardiovascular Anesthesiologists; Society for Cardiovascular Angiography and Interventions; Society of Interventional Radiology; Society of Thoracic Surgeons; Society for Vascular Medicine. 2010 ACCF/AHA/AATS/ACR/ASA/SCA/SCAI/SIR/STS/SVM guidelines for the diagnosis and management of patients with Thoracic Aortic Disease: a report of the American College of Cardiology Foundation/American Heart Association Task Force on Practice Guidelines, American Association for Thoracic Surgery, American College of Radiology, American Stroke Association, Society of Cardiovascular Anesthesiologists, Society for Cardiovascular

Angiography and Interventions, Society of Interventional Radiology, Society of Thoracic Surgeons, and Society for Vascular Medicine. Circulation. 2010;121(13):e266–369.

3. Hagan PG, Nienaber CA, Isselbacher EM, Bruckman D, Karavite DJ, Russman PL, Evangelista A, Fattori R, Suzuki T, Oh JK, Moore AG, Malouf JF, Pape LA, Gaca C, Sechtem U, Lenferink S, Deutsch HJ, Diedrichs H, Marcos y Robles J, Llovet A, Gilon D, Das SK, Armstrong WF, Deeb GM, Eagle KA. The International Registry of Acute Aortic Dissection (IRAD): new insights into an old disease. JAMA. 2000;283(7):897–903.

4. Svensson LG, Kouchoukos NT, Miller DC, Bavaria JE, Coselli JS, Curi MA, Eggebrecht H, Elefteriades JA, Erbel R, Gleason TG, Lytle BW, Mitchell RS, Nienaber CA, Roselli EE, Safi HJ, Shemin RJ, Sicard GA, Sundt 3rd TM, Szeto WY, Wheatley 3rd GH, Society of Thoracic Surgeons Endovascular Surgery Task Force. Expert consensus document on the treatment of descending thoracic aortic disease using endovascular stent-grafts. Ann Thorac Surg. 2008;85:S1–41.

5. Gilon D, Mehta RH, Oh JK, Januzzi Jr JL, Bossone E, Cooper JV, Smith DE, Fang J, Nienaber CA, Eagle KA, Isselbacher EM, International Registry of Acute Aortic Dissection Group. Characteristics and in-hospital outcomes of patients with cardiac tamponade complicating type A acute aortic dissection. Am J Cardiol. 2009;103:1029–31.

6. Gaul C, Dietrich W, Friedrich I, Sirch J, Erbguth FJ. Neurological symptoms in type A aortic dissections. Stroke. 2007;38:292–7.

7. Akin I, Kische S, Ince H, Nienaber CA. Indication, timing and results of endovascular treatment of type B dissection. Eur J Vasc Endovasc Surg. 2009;37:289–96.

8. Trimarchi S, Eagle KA, Nienaber CA, Pyeritz RE, Jonker FH, Suzuki T, O'Gara PT, Hutchinson SJ, Rampoldi V, Grassi V, Bossone E, Muhs BE, Evangelista A, Tsai TT, Froehlich JB, Cooper JV, Montgomery D, Meinhardt G, Myrmel T, Upchurch GR, Sundt TM, Isselbacher EM. Importance of refractory pain and hypertension inacute type B aortic dissection: insights from the International Registry of Acute Aortic Dissection (IRAD). Circulation. 2010;122:1283–9.

9. Kitai T, Kaji S, Yamamuro A, Tani T, Tamita K, Kinoshita M, Ehara N, Kobori A, Nasu M, Okada Y, Furukawa Y. Clinical outcomes of medical therapy and timely operation in initially diagnosed type a aortic intramural hematoma: a 20-year experience. Circulation. 2009;120(11 Suppl):S292–8.

10. Evangelista A, Dominguez R, Sebastia C, Salas A, Permanyer-Miralda G, Avegliano G, Gomez-Bosh Z, Gonzalez-Alujas T, Garcia del Castillo H, Soler-Soler J. Prognostic value of clinical and morphologic findings in short-term evolution of aortic intramural haematoma. Therapeutic implications. Eur Heart J. 2004;25(1):81–7.

11. von Kodolitsch Y, Csösz SK, Koschyk DH, Schalwat I, Loose R, Karck M, Dieckmann C, Fattori R, Haverich A, Berger J, Meinertz T, Nienaber CA. Intramural hematoma of the aorta: predictors of progression to dissection and rupture. Circulation. 2003;107(8):1158–63.

12. Tsai TT, Evangelista A, Nienaber CA, Trimarchi S, Sechtem U, Fattori R, Myrmel T, Pape L, Cooper JV, Smith DE, Fang J, Isselbacher E, Eagle KA, International Registry of Acute Aortic Dissection (IRAD). Long-term survival in patients presenting with type A acute aortic dissection: insights from the International Registry of Acute Aortic Dissection (IRAD). Circulation. 2006;114(1 Suppl):I350–6.

13. Tsai TT, Fattori R, Trimarchi S, Isselbacher E, Myrmel T, Evangelista A, Hutchison S, Sechtem U, Cooper JV, Smith DE, Pape L, Froehlich J, Raghupathy A, Januzzi JL, Eagle KA, Nienaber CA, International Registry of Acute Aortic Dissection. Long-term survival in patients presenting with type B acute aortic dissection: insights from the International Registry of Acute Aortic Dissection. Circulation. 2006;114(21):2226–31.

14. Evangelista A, Dominguez R, Sebastia C, Salas A, Permanyer-Miralda G, Avegliano G, Elorz C, Gonzalez-Alujas T, Garcia Del Castillo H, Soler-Soler J. Long-term follow-up of aortic intramural hematoma: predictors of outcome. Circulation. 2003;108(5):583–9.

15. Gysi J, Schaffner T, Mohacsi P, Aeschbacher B, Althaus U, Carrel T. Early and late outcome of operated and non-operated acute dissection of the descending aorta. Eur J Cardiothorac Surg. 1997;11:1163–9; discussion 1169–70.

16. Yu H-Y, Chen Y-S, Huang S-C, Wang S-S, Lin F-Y. Late outcome of patients with aortic dissection: study of a national database. Eur J Cardiothorac Surg. 2004;25:683–90.

17. Junoven T, Ergin MA, Galla JC, Lansman SI, McCullough JN, Nguyen K, Bodian CA, Ehrlich MP, Spielvogel D, Klein JJ, Griepp RB. Risk factors for rupture of chronic type B dissections. J Thorac Cardiovasc Surg. 1999;117:776–86.

18. Halstead JC, Chir B, Meier M, Etz C, Spielvogel D, Bodial C, Wurm M, Shahani R, Griepp RB. The fate of the distal

aorta after repair of acute type A aortic dissection. J Thorac Cardiovasc Surg. 2007;133:127–35.

19. Tsai TT, Evangelista A, Nienaber CA, Myrmel T, Meinhardt G, Cooper JV, Smith DE, Suzuki T, Fattori R, Llovet A, Froehlich J, Hutchison S, Distante A, Sundt T, Beckman J, Januzzi JL, Isselbacher EM, Eagle KA. Partial thrombosis of the false lumen in patients with acute type B aortic dissection. N Engl J Med. 2007;357:349–59.

20. Umaña JP, Lai DT, Mitchell RS, Moore KA, Rodriguez F, Robbins RC, Oyer PE, Dake MD, Shumway NE, Reitz BA, Miller DC. Is medical therapy still the optimal treatment strategy for patients with acute type B aortic dissections? J Thorac Cardiovasc Surg. 2002;124:896–910.

21. Song JM, Kim SD, Kim JH, Kim MJ, Kang DH, Seo JB, Lim TH, Lee JW, Song MG, Song JK. Long-term predictors of descending aorta aneurismal change in patients with aortic dissection. J Am Coll Cardiol. 2007;50:799–804.

22. Hata M, Sezai A, Niino T, Yoda M, Wakui S, Unosawa S, Umeda T, Shimura K, Osaka S, Furukawa N, Kimura H, Minami K. Prognosis for patients with type B acute aortic dissection. Risk analysis of early death and requirement for elective surgery. Circ J. 2007;71:1279–82.

23. Evangelista A, Salas A, Ribera A, Ferreira-González I, Cuellar H, Pineda V, González-Alujas T, Bijnens B, Permanyer-Miralda G, Garcia-Dorado D. Long-term outcome of aortic dissection with patent false lumen: predictive role of entry tear size and location. Circulation. 2012;125(25):3133–41.

24. Kimura N, Tanaka M, Kawahito K, Yamaguchi A, Ino T, Adachi H. Influence of patent false lumen on long-term outcome after surgery for acute type A aortic dissection. J Thorac Cardiovasc Surg. 2008;136:1160–6.

25. Fattouch K, Sampognaro R, Navarra E, Caruso M, Pisano C, Coppola G, Speziale G, Ruvolo G. Long-term results after repair of type A acute aortic dissection according to false lumen patency. Ann Thorac Surg. 2009;88:1244–50.

26. Baliga RR, Nienaber CA, Bossone E, Oh JK, Isselbacher EM, Sechtem U, Fattori R, Raman SV, Eagle KA. The role of imaging in aortic dissection and related syndromes. JACC Cardiovasc Imaging. 2014;7(4):406–24.

27. Erbel R, Alfonso F, Boileau C, Dirsch O, Eber B, Haverich A, Rakowski H, Struyven J, Radegran K, Sechtem U, Taylor J, Zollikofer C, Klein WW, Mulder B, Providencia LA, Task

258   E. Bossone et al.

Force on Aortic Dissection, European Society of Cardiology. Diagnosis and management of aortic dissection. Eur Heart J. 2001;22(18):1642–81.

28. Booher AM, Eagle KA, Bossone E. Acute aortic syndromes. Herz. 2011;36(6):480–7.

29. Bossone E, Suzuki T, Eagle KA, Weinsaft JW. Diagnosis of acute aortic syndromes: imaging and beyond. Herz. 2013;38(3):269–76.

30. Suzuki T, Bossone E, Sawaki D, Jánosi RA, Erbel R, Eagle K, Nagai R. Biomarkers of aortic diseases. Am Heart J. 2013;165(1):15–25.

31. Tahara N, Kai H, Yamagishi S, Mizoguchi M, Nakaura H, Ishibashi M, Kaida H, Baba K, Hayabuchi N, Imaizumi T. Vascular inflammation evaluated by [18 F]-fluorodeoxyglucose positron emission tomography is associated with the metabolic syndrome. J Am Coll Cardiol. 2007;49(14):1533–9.

32. Reeps C, Pelisek J, Bundschuh RA, Gurdan M, Zimmermann A, Ockert S, Dobritz M, Eckstein HH, Essler M. Imaging of acute and chronic aortic dissection by 18 F-FDG PET/CT. J Nucl Med. 2010;51(5):686–91.

33. Sangiorgi G, Trimarchi S, Mauriello A, Righini P, Bossone E, Suzuki T, Rampoldi V, Eagle KA. Plasma levels of metalloproteinases-9 and –2 in the acute and subacute phases of type A and type B aortic dissection. J Cardiovasc Med (Hagerstown). 2006;7(5):307–15.

34. Chan KK, Rabkin SW. Increasing prevalence of hypertension among patients with thoracic aorta dissection: trends over eight decades – a structured meta-analysis. Am J Hypertens. 2014;27(7):907–17.

35. Mancia G, Fagard R, Narkiewicz K, Redon J, Zanchetti A, Böhm M, Christiaens T, Cifkova R, De Backer G, Dominiczak A, Galderisi M, Grobbee DE, Jaarsma T, Kirchhof P, Kjeldsen SE, Laurent S, Manolis AJ, Nilsson PM, Ruilope LM, Schmieder RE, Sirnes PA, Sleight P, Viigimaa M, Waeber B, Zannad F, Redon J, Dominiczak A, Narkiewicz K, Nilsson PM, Burnier M, Viigimaa M, Ambrosioni E, Caufield M, Coca A, Olsen MH, Schmieder RE, Tsioufis C, van de Borne P, Zamorano JL, Achenbach S, Baumgartner H, Bax JJ, Bueno H, Dean V, Deaton C, Erol C, Fagard R, Ferrari R, Hasdai D, Hoes AW, Kirchhof P, Knuuti J, Kolh P, Lancellotti P, Linhart A, Nihoyannopoulos P, Piepoli MF, Ponikowski P, Sirnes PA, Tamargo JL, Tendera M, Torbicki A, Wijns W, Windecker S, Clement DL, Coca A, Gillebert TC, Tendera M, Rosei EA, Ambrosioni E, Anker SD, Bauersachs J, Hitij JB, Caulfield M, De Buyzere M, De Geest S, Derumeaux

GA, Erdine S, Farsang C, Funck-Brentano C, Gerc V, Germano G, Gielen S, Haller H, Hoes AW, Jordan J, Kahan T, Komajda M, Lovic D, Mahrholdt H, Olsen MH, Ostergren J, Parati G, Perk J, Polonia J, Popescu BA, Reiner Z, Rydén L, Sirenko Y, Stanton A, Struijker-Boudier H, Tsioufis C, van de Borne P, Vlachopoulos C, Volpe M, Wood DA. 2013 ESH/ESC guidelines for the management of arterial hypertension: the Task Force for the Management of Arterial Hypertension of the European Society of Hypertension (ESH) and of the European Society of Cardiology (ESC). Eur Heart J. 2013;34(28):2159–219.

36. Ong KT, Perdu J, De Backer J, Bozec E, Collignon P, Emmerich J, Fauret al, Fiessinger JN, Germain DP, Georgesco G, Hulot JS, De Paepe A, Plauchu H, Jeunemaitre X, Laurent S, Boutouyrie P. Effect of celiprolol on prevention of cardiovascular events in vascular Ehlers-Danlos syndrome: a prospective randomised, open, blinded-endpoints trial. Lancet. 2010;376(9751):1476–84.

37. Shores J, Berger KR, Murphy EA, Pyeritz RE. Progression of aortic dilatation and the benefit of long-term beta-adrenergic blockade in Marfan's syndrome. N Engl J Med. 1994;330(19):1335–41.

38. Golledge J, Eagle KA. Acute aortic dissection. Lancet. 2008;372(9632):55–66.

39. Suzuki T, Isselbacher EM, Nienaber CA, Pyeritz RE, Eagle KA, Tsai TT, Cooper JV, Januzzi Jr JL, Braverman AC, Montgomery DG, Fattori R, Pape L, Harris KM, Booher A, Oh JK, Peterson M, Ramanath VS, Froehlich JB, IRAD Investigators. Type-selective benefits of medications in treatment of acute aortic dissection (from the International Registry of Acute Aortic Dissection [IRAD]). Am J Cardiol. 2012;109(1):122–7.

40. Genoni M, Paul M, Jenni R, Graves K, Seifert B, Turina M. Chronic beta-blocker therapy improves outcome and reduces treatment costs in chronic type B aortic dissection. Eur J Cardiothorac Surg. 2001;19(5):606–10.

41. Ganaha F, Miller DC, Sugimoto K, Do YS, Minamiguchi H, Saito H, Mitchell RS, Dake MD. The prognosis of aortic intramural hematoma with and without penetrating atherosclerose ulcer: a clinical and radiological analysis. Circulation. 2002;106:342–8.

42. Finkbohner R, Johnston D, Crawford ES, Coselli J, Milewicz DM. Marfan syndrome: long-term survival and complications after aortic aneurysm repair. Circulation. 1995;91:728–33.

43. Silverman DI, Burton KJ, Gray J, Bosner MS, Kouchoukos NT, Roman MJ, Boxer M, Devereux RB, Tsipouras P. Life expectancy in the Marfan syndrome. Am J Cardiol. 1995;75:157–60.

44. Umana JP, Miller DC, Mitchell RS. What is the best treatment for patients with acute type B aortic dissections – medical, surgical, or endovascular stentgrafting? Ann Thorac Surg. 2002;74(5):S1840–3; discussion S57–63.

45. Mochizuki S, Dahlöf B, Shimizu M, Ikewaki K, Yoshikawa M, Taniguchi I, Ohta M, Yamada T, Ogawa K, Kanae K, Kawai M, Seki S, Okazaki F, Taniguchi M, Yoshida S, Tajima N, Jikei Heart Study Group. Valsartan in a Japanese population with hypertension and other cardiovascular disease (Jikei Heart Study): a randomised, open-label, blinded end point morbidity-mortality study. Lancet. 2007;369(9571):1431–9.

46. Brooke BS, Habashi JP, Judge DP, Patel N, Loeys B, Dietz HC. Angiotensin II blockade and aortic-root dilation in Marfan's syndrome. N Engl J Med. 2008;358(26):2787–95.

47. Groenink M, den Hartog AW, Franken R, Radonic T, de Waard V, Timmermans J, Scholte AJ, van den Berg MP, Spijkerboer AM, Marquering HA, Zwinderman AH, Mulder BJ. Losartan reduces aortic dilatation rate in adults with Marfan syndrome: a randomized controlled trial. Eur Heart J. 2013;34(45):3491–500.

48. Ahimastos AA, Aggarwal A, D'Orsa KM, Formosa MF, White AJ, Savarirayan R, Dart AM, Kingwell BA. Effect of perindopril on large artery stiffness and aortic root diameter in patients with Marfan syndrome: a randomized controlled trial. JAMA. 2007;298(13):1539–47.

49. Mukherjee D, Januzzi JL. Long-term medical therapy in aortic dissection. In: Aortic dissection and related syndromes. New York: Springer; 2007.

50. Sakakura K, Kubo N, Ako J, Fujiwara N, Funayama H, Ikeda N, Nakamura T, Sugawara Y, Yasu T, Kawakami M, Momomura S. Determinants of long-term mortality in patients with type B acute aortic dissection. Am J Hypertens. 2009;22:371–7.

51. Chan KK, Lai P, Wright JM. First-line beta-blockers versus other antihypertensive medications for chronic type B aortic dissection. Cochrane Database Syst Rev. 2014;2:CD010426. doi: 10.1002/14651858.CD010426.pub2.

52. Hirsch AT, Haskal ZJ, Hertzer NR, Bakal CW, Creager MA, Halperin JL, Hiratzka LF, Murphy WR, Olin JW, Puschett JB, Rosenfield KA, Sacks D, Stanley JC, Taylor Jr LM, White CJ, White J, White RA, Antman EM, Smith Jr SC, Adams CD, Anderson JL, Faxon DP, Fuster V, Gibbons RJ, Hunt SA, Jacobs AK, Nishimura R, Ornato JP, Page RL, Riegel B, American Association for Vascular Surgery; Society for

Vascular Surgery; Society for Cardiovascular Angiography and Interventions; Society for Vascular Medicine and Biology; Society of Interventional Radiology; ACC/AHA Task Force on Practice Guidelines Writing Committee to Develop Guidelines for the Management of Patients With Peripheral Arterial Disease; American Association of Cardiovascular and Pulmonary Rehabilitation; National Heart, Lung, and Blood Institute; Society for Vascular Nursing; Trans Atlantic Inter-Society Consensus; Vascular Disease Foundation. ACC/AHA 2005 Practice Guidelines for the management of patients with peripheral arterial disease (lower extremity, renal, mesenteric, and abdominal aortic). Circulation. 2006;113:e463–654.

53. Tazaki J, Morimoto T, Sakata R, Okabayashi H, Yamazaki F, Nishiwaki N, Mitsudo K, Kimura T, the CREDO-Kyoto PCI/CABG Registry Cohort-2 Investigators. Impact of statin therapy on patients with coronary heart disease and aortic aneurysm or dissection. J Vasc Surg. 2014;2.

54. Song SW, Yoo KJ, Kim DK, Cho BK, Yi G, Chang BC. Effects of early anticoagulation on the degree of thrombosis. After repair of acute DeBakey type I aortic dissection. Ann Thorac Surg. 2011;92(4):1367–74; discussion 1374–5.

55. Cañadas MV, Vilacosta I, Ferreirós J, Bustos A, Díaz-Mediavilla J, Rodríguez E. Intramural aortic hematoma and anticoagulation. Rev Esp Cardiol. 2007;60(2):201–4.

56. Ockene IS, Miller NH. Cigarette smoking, cardiovascular disease, and stroke: a statement for healthcare professionals from the American Heart Association. American Heart Association Task Force on Risk Reduction. Circulation. 1997;96:3243–7.

57. Daly LE, Mulcahy R, Graham IM, Hickey N. Long term effect on mortality of stopping smoking after unstable angina and myocardial infarction. Br Med J (Clin Res Ed). 1983;287:324–6.

58. U.S. Department of Health and Human Services, Public Health Service Agency. Clinical Practice Guidelines: Number 18. Smoking Cessation 1996; AHCPR Publication 96–0692.

59. Dapunt OE, Galla JD, Sadeghi AM, Lansman SL, Mezrow CK, de Asla RA, Quintana C, Wallenstein S, Ergin AM, Griepp RB. The natural history of thoracic aortic aneurysms. J Thorac Cardiovasc Surg. 1994;107:1323–32.

60. Griepp RB, Ergin MA, Galla JD, Lansman SL, McCullough JN, Nguyen KH, Klein JJ, Spielvogel D. Natural history of

descending thoracic and thoracoabdominal aneurysms. Ann Thorac Surg. 1999;67:1927–30.
61. Fattori R, Cao P, De Rango P, Czerny M, Evangelista A, Nienaber C, Rousseau H, Schepens M. Interdisciplinary expert consensus document on management of type B aortic dissection. J Am Coll Cardiol. 2013;61(16):1661–78.

Index

A. Evangelista, C.A. Nienaber (eds.), *Pharmacotherapy
in Aortic Disease*, Current Cardiovascular Therapy, Vol. 7,
DOI 10.1007/978-3-319-09555-4,
© Springer International Publishing Switzerland 2015

266   Index